CHIROPRACTIC REVEALED

One on One with the Great Masters of a Misunderstood Profession

DAVID K. SCHEINER, D.C.

Foreword by Reggie Gold, D.C., Ph.C.

SCRIBE
DOC
PUBLICATIONS, INC.

CHIROPRACTIC REVEALED
One on One with the
Great Masters of a
Misunderstood Profession

Published by:
Scribe Doc Publications, Inc.
P. O. Box 71524
Marietta, GA 30007

Copyright © 2009 by David K. Scheiner, D.C.

All rights reserved. This publication may not be reproduced, stored in a retrieval system, or trasmitted in whole or in part, in any form or by any means, electronic, mechanical, photocopying, recording, or otherwise, without prior written permission of the author and publisher.

ISBN: 978-0-9842082-0-3

First Printing: September 2009
Printed in the United States of America

Additional copies of this book may be ordered
by calling 678-920-8484
Website: www.ChiropracticRevealed.com

Design by Marty Marsh, www.martymarsh.com

All photographs are used with the permission
of the respective copyright holders.

"*The questions probe the very heart of what's happening in chiropractic today! A 'must read' book for every D.C. who cares about the profession and the future of chiropractic.*" — Arno Burnier, D.C., Founder of Masterpiece Seminars, Cafe of Life, and Zeechi

"*Dr. David Scheiner managed to get some of the top chiropractic leaders to talk candidly about many of the most important topics facing our profession.*" — Pasquale J. Cerasoli, D.C., pioneering chiropractor since 1947 and post graduate instructor

"*A wonderful collection of intriguing chiropractic figures brought together for one book. Their answers will spark debate, hope, and intrigue.*" — Gerard Clum, D.C., president of Life Chiropractic College West

"*Inspiring stories, enlightening principles, and time-tested actions that will help chiropractors serve even more millions of patients.*" — John F. Demartini, D.C., bestselling author of "Count Your Blessings" and contributor to "The Secret"

"*Absolutely compelling! It's like sitting in a room full of chiropractic legends. Amazing stuff.*" — Thom Gelardi, D.C., founder and past president of Sherman College of Straight Chiropractic

"*Kudos to Dr. Scheiner for bringing together, in one place, the insights of some of chiropractic's greatest minds.*" — Christopher Kent, D.C., J.D., co-founder of Chiropractic Leadership Alliance

"*A perfect blend of fascinating personal details and astute professional observations.*" — Fabrizio Mancini, D.C., president of Parker College of Chiropractic

"*A printed Mastermind Meeting! Chock full of concepts and visions — sure to inspire you with the wisdom to build a life of significance.*" — Larry Markson, D.C., founder of The Markson Connection

"*Reading these chiropractors' experiences connects us to our roots, rekindles our passion and inspires our vision for the future of chiropractic.*" — Jeanne Ohm, D.C., founder of "Makin' Miracles... Connecting Kids & Chiropractic"

"You hold in your hands a 'must read' chiropractic manual collected from the best and the brightest minds in the profession. Dr. Scheiner's interviews probe and dissect the consciousness that drives them. This brilliant anthology is jam-packed with the clues needed to understand the intricacies and dynamics of this awesome thing we call chiropractic! Invest your time reading it — you're worth it." — Tony Palermo, D.C., Founder/CEO: Get Back to Basics (Success Coaching and Consulting)

"Dr. Scheiner's book is an incredible compilation of insights and stories from chiropractic leaders and legends. I am amazed by the wisdom and passion that leaps out from every page. This should be required reading for every D.C. and student!" — Terry A. Rondberg, D.C., founder and CEO of the World Chiropractic Alliance, and publisher of The Chiropractic Journal

"This is a great book that intertwines personalities, chiropractic history and principles into a marvelous readable style. It is a must read for every chiropractor, student, patient, or retired D.C." — Armand Rossi, D.C., famed worldwide lecturer on pediatric chiropractic

"This book realizes the famous and near famous men and women of the great chiropractic life." — James Sigafoose, D.C., team teacher with Parker Seminars for 15 years and Dynamic Essentials for more than 45 years

"A great balance of interesting personal history and profound professional insights." – Guy Riekeman, D.C., president, Life University

"It's nice to think the universe will open up, but sometimes it needs a crowbar to help it. This fascinating volume is that crowbar, opening up a universe of insights and knowledge that can ultimately change the course of chiropractic's future." – Reggie Gold, D.C., Ph.C., chiropractic legend, philosopher, and teacher

"A current perspective from leaders who've influenced the development of chiropractic and will inspire future chiropractors to continue carrying this legacy." – Claudia Anrig, D.C., Founder of Peter Pan Potential

Contents

Dedication

To my mom, who left us too soon, told me to always follow my heart, and to someday write a book.

About the Author

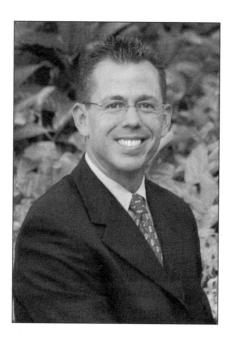

*E*ven before he graduated Life University in 1996, **David K. Scheiner, D.C.,** had a strong desire to find ways to more fully express life and wholeness, both physically and spiritually — and to help others reach that same goal. Chiropractic allowed him to realize that aspiration.

During his 12 years in private practice, David owned and operated three successful chiropractic offices in and around Atlanta before taking his passion for chiropractic and the human cause to the next level. Because he feels strongly that every person has the right to have a nervous system clear of interference, his mission now is to bring the true chiropractic message to the world through his writing and lectures.

He and his family live in Atlanta.

Foreword

By Reggie Gold, D.C., Ph.C.

More than a century has passed since its founding, and the chiropractic profession appears to be still tangled up in philosophical intricacies and disrupted by internal squabbling. The inevitable result? Its roots have been confused and obscured.

Yet, how can one truly understand chiropractic until the factors that blended together to create its history are known? It's not possible.

Chiropractic as it is today is the result of the way chiropractors themselves have viewed their profession. With the publishing of this book, David Scheiner has given us the opportunity to gain valuable insights into the experiences and opinions of some of chiropractic's legendary pioneers and best-known figures.

Sharing such vital information isn't just an interesting and leisurely stroll into the past. We can't hope to improve and advance chiropractic unless we strive to fight less, know one another better, and love a whole lot more. Without question, chiropractic needs more forgiving and chiropractors need to be more "for giving."

It's nice to think the universe will open up, but sometimes it needs a crowbar to help it. This fascinating volume *is* that crowbar, opening up a universe of insights and knowledge that can ultimately change the course of chiropractic's future.

Introduction

Throughout our lives, the universe presents us with wondrous gifts. Yet often, before a gift is ever unwrapped and opened, we assume we know what's inside the box and use that illusory version of the true gift instead of what's really there.

"Chiropractic Revealed" is an opportunity as well as a book. It's an opportunity to take a gift that was provided to each one of us and open it in order to discover the truth behind what it is we call *chiropractic*.

Most people engaged in the chiropractic profession have wondered why chiropractic is so misunderstood even among those involved in it and why the public at large doesn't understand what chiropractors do.

This book will answer the questions our profession has faced for so long: "Why can't we all just get along and stop the internal fighting?" and "When will the general public understand what it is that we truly do and see us in our accurate framework?"

When you're in the forest and the wind meanders through the trees, what's the reason you aren't able to hear the messages the universe is sharing with you through the sounds of the rustling leaves and rattling branches? It's speaking right at you and yet you can't hear what it's saying.

While the messages and metaphors are always there for us to decipher, analyze, and learn, our educated minds get in the way — preventing the universal messages from making their useful and necessary imprints on our nervous systems and genetic coding. Often we're afraid people won't understand the truth about what we have to offer them, and since the ego is always trying to have us "look good," we succumb to fear and provide some watered down version of the Grand Prize.

D.D. Palmer presented chiropractic to us and his son, B.J., packaged it in a way he thought chiropractors, students, and the lay public would understand, in the context of what was available and occurring at the time. It's quite possible the whole paradigm has been presented incorrectly all along!

Had it been developed and promoted in conjunction with the constructive energies and forces of the universe, the wonderful gift we call chiropractic would have been unwrapped and presented fittingly. Many more people would be wearing the entire chiropractic wardrobe than are putting it on today.

Now, we have the chance to give the gift anew!

In this book, you'll hear from the Great Masters of our chiropractic profession. Through their stories, opinions, and truths, they've laid the groundwork for us to take chiropractic to the masses so that every adult and child can experience its wonderful benefits.

Each chapter presents an electrifying tale about where chiropractic may have gone astray, what it must do to get back on track, and how chiropractic will ultimately enable the whole planet to experience an enhanced quality of existence! The time has certainly come for the world to experience chiropractic as it never has before.

At this very moment, the universe is presenting us with a window of opportunity that will be open for only a short period of time. It is within this time that our voices and messages of truth can and must be heard. Our very livelihood and human existence depend on it.

Take your copy of this wonderful mastermind compilation in hand, sit in your favorite place, and journey with me so that together we can go one on one with the Great Masters of this misunderstood profession we call CHIROPRACTIC!

With much love and appreciation I give my present to you — "Chiropractic Revealed."

David K. Scheiner, D.C.

Claudia Anrig

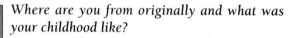

Where are you from originally and what was your childhood like?

I'm originally from Dearborn, Michigan. My parents emigrated from Switzerland but we three kids were born in Dearborn. When my dad entered chiropractic college, we moved to the West Coast for the rest of our lives. I call Fresno, California home now.

Childhood was fabulous and I was very fortunate to have great, loving parents who are still alive. One of the things they taught us was that whatever you put your mind to, you can achieve — there's no limit to the goals you can set in your life. They did say it would take work, though. I was given this huge opportunity to think big as a child and was never brought up with any limitations, just to be good at whatever I decided to do.

What inspired you to get involved with chiropractic?

Now this is an interesting tale. My mom is one of those chiropractic miracle stories we hear about. When she was pregnant with my younger sister, Susi, she couldn't walk because of lower back pain, so she went the medical route. Doctors told her that once she gave birth, the pain would ease up. She gave birth and the pain just got worse. At that point, the medical profession basically told her to learn how to crawl and bear weight as little as possible.

This went on for months and my dad ended up working all day and being Mr. Mom as well. While at the grocery store one day, the gentleman at the counter said, "Gosh we haven't seen your wife and kids for a while, is everything okay?"

My dad, who's normally a real quiet man, shared what was happening to my mom, and the man said immediately, "She has to go see a chiropractor." Back then, my parents couldn't even pronounce the word, let alone spell it. Yet, they were looking for something called hope, so they went to the chiropractor the next day. He X-rayed, examined, and began adjusting my mom and within a few weeks she was out of pain. A few weeks later, she could walk again so she stopped going.

We moved to Arizona because my parents were tired of shoveling that white stuff called snow. About a year and a half later, my mom started having her old problem again because, as all chiropractors know, most people don't understand they have to stay with adjustments even when there's no pain.

Thanks to the chiropractor's explanations, and the health care class he gave, my parents realized that, since my mom's problem could have begun in childhood, they should bring their children in for care.

My mom had deteriorated horribly so she decided to go to a chiropractor, since the first one helped so much. This one again X-rayed, examined, and began adjusting her and within a few weeks she was walking again, pain free.

But there was a really big difference in the two chiropractic experiences. Both got results but the second chiropractor was more education-oriented. He told my mom she had phase-two to phase-three spinal degeneration in her early 30s. When she was a child, she had back pain and leg cramps, which everyone just called growing pains. This developed into other issues as a young woman.

Thanks to the chiropractor's explanations, and the health care class he gave, my parents realized that, since my mom's problem could have begun in childhood, they should bring their children in for care.

My first chiropractic adjustment was between the ages of 5 and 6. From 6 to 7, whenever my parents asked me what I wanted for my birthday, my answer was a full spine X-ray series, so I could take them to school and give a lay lecture about why all children needed chiropractic care.

Dr. Guest, my chiropractor at that time, thought that was such a fabulous wish he gave me those X-rays as a birthday gift. I took them to school and gave the class a three-day lay lecture on the benefits of chiropractic care!

I knew even at this young age that my mission was to be a chiropractor. My dad had the same thought and we moved to Los Angeles, where he enrolled in Cleveland College. Quite often back then, classes were held in an old house and the garage was the cadaver room. They offered both day and night school at that time, so my dad worked during the day and went to school in the evening hours.

Once in awhile, a Friday "date night" with my dad consisted of going to classes with him. Chemistry was a lot easier back then than it was when I went to college! It was a really great time and I loved chiropractic as a kid. I loved going to the seminars with my parents; the whole family would sit in the front row with a pad and pen and take notes. My brother Daniel and my sister Susi are chiropractors now as well. We practiced together up until two years ago, when my sister moved to Florida. We had a family practice all together and my mom was the office manager. It's really in our family blood and it spans two generations.

Where do you currently reside and how are you spending your time these days?

I live in Fresno, California and I keep quite busy. I don't cook and — God bless my husband — I married somebody who is wonderful and takes on that chore. I'm still in full-time practice, not a semi-retirement practice. I have been in full-time practice now for about 27 years and part of my joy is mentoring other chiropractors.

I started what I call "Generations" six years ago. It gives me satisfaction nurturing younger doctors or doctors who have been plateaued. That was a really important part of my life and I continue to teach 25 weeks out of the year. I still do mentoring two days a week and — somewhere within all of this — I still have that creative bug in me to write and produce educational materials.

Right now, I'm in the mid-portion of editing the second edition of my textbook, "Pediatric Chiropractic." I don't really have free time, although I can actually read a book while I'm sitting on the airplane going from point A to point B. I am so pleased with the textbook because I remember how, when I was in school, textbooks weren't around and we had to learn things like this from seminars and stories.

Honestly, when I went through chiropractic college, I didn't learn how to examine or adjust a child. I wasn't taught any of that! I knew, from being adjusted as a kid, that chiropractic was for everybody. The textbook I wrote was important because both students and doctors could finally have a reference book that would help them provide better care from prenatal, to newborn, and to adolescence.

How does the profession differ now from when you first became involved?

We can easily spend two hours on this one. One thing is that the philosophy, although alive and well on many chiropractic campuses, is being taught more from an historical point of view rather than for the purpose of living the philosophy and principles. We happen to be a profession whose roots and essence are within that philosophy.

What I am also seeing is that, because of that lack of teaching (perhaps they think it's ancient and archaic) many chiropractic students have never really had the kind of personal experience with chiropractic that brought many of us to it as a career. I see a lot of young doctors moving into chiropractic as a health profession, not a lifestyle with a mission to go out there and really change the world.

Of course, I also see the political move to dictate that our profession should stay in the "symptom relief model." That's why so many of us are saying we need to honor relief-based care but we definitely need room for the wellness and prevention models to be out there.

Wellness and prevention are really the essence of chiropractic and we need to focus on that if we are to survive and be the profession we should be in the next 100 years. If we're not embracing wellness, we have totally missed the whole opportunity D.D. and B.J. Palmer gave us.

We have done relief care real well for the last 100 years and the next 100 had better be in the wellness area where every mother, father, and child is receiving chiropractic care.

Our role is to educate future generations that they should wake up every day understanding that receiving chiropractic care is just like preventive dental care. It's part of a person's lifestyle. One of my hopes is that chiropractic will be incorporated in a normal lifestyle and people won't think twice about whether or not they need to bring their kids to a chiropractor. It will be their lifestyle and they'll automatically bring them in. That's my hope for wellness.

How does chiropractic relate to a person realizing his or her fullest human potential?

When we look at human potential, everybody has their own imprint. You can call it their hard-wiring — who they are and how they're going to express themselves. If we, as chiropractors, can eliminate the interference to that potential, we act as facilitators for the individual's journey in life. We're very blessed that we can eliminate interference, and through teaching, educating, and acting as lifestyle teachers, we can also enhance the human potential of others.

How do chiropractic and performance relate?

Anytime you improve quality of life by eliminating or minimizing interference, performance on physical, emotional, and spiritual levels is also enhanced. Here we get to see people realizing their full expression.

If we look at children from an anatomical point of view and in relation to performance, having their spines checked for vertebral subluxation is paramount because they are going through developmental milestones. The first year of life is dramatic and thereafter through adolescence we need to check for the presence of vertebral subluxation and eliminate that interference through the chiropractic adjustment.

What we're offering children in the developmental years is huge and more powerful than during any other stage of life. What we do in the first 5, 10, and 18 years is vital and can allow these kids to ultimately enjoy a stronger immune system and, on a personal level, a better mind-body awareness. Even their spirituality will be at its best expression.

The first year of life is dramatic and thereafter through adolescence we need to check for the presence of vertebral subluxation and eliminate that interference through the chiropractic adjustment.

We know that one of the benefits enjoyed by pregnant women under chiropractic care is that they express little or no morning sickness and function at a very high level in the first, second, and third trimester. They report to us constantly a reduction of aches, pains, and discomfort and also notice a marked increase in energy.

The feedback they give us tells of overall enhanced quality of life and they feel they made a good decision by seeking chiropractic. As far as labor and delivery are concerned, one of the things we know is that a specific sacral adjustment will produce a stronger likelihood of the fetus being in a head-down vertex position, which means shorter labor, shorter delivery time, and less need for invasive techniques by orthodox medicine.

The availability of chiropractic care for the first and second trimester is critical because we see decreased birth injuries and safer deliveries. Although we have no research on this, chiropractors who have expansive prenatal practices report that newborns right out of the birth canal have a stronger neck and hold their heads upright. Also, their eyes immediately track when they hear voices in the room. That's actually a developmental stage that shouldn't be happening until 8 to 12 weeks later — and it's happening right after birth! The interesting thing is that we're not even doing fetal adjustments but what we're doing with the mother makes a huge difference in the infant.

How does chiropractic offer people an opportunity to realize an enhanced quality of life?

Individuals need to understand what quality of life is. For a person enduring a chronic pattern of pain, any improvement is certainly better than nothing. If they come into chiropractic care, you can't promise them that they will be 100 percent better, but you can give them something we call hope. Quality of life is that ability to wake up every day and just feel like you are grounded on a physical, mental, and emotional level.

What do you feel has happened to the chiropractic profession that may have limited it from being seen by the world in its true nature?

We got stuck in the pain and symptom-relief model. Although that's important in that we're helping those who are suffering, we have failed to educate people that we also stand for wellness and prevention.

Many chiropractors, possibly a silent majority of the profession, have been practicing wellness, although we haven't had a strong voice. On the political level, everyone focused on rights for the relief-care model in chiropractic rather than supporting those who provide wellness and prevention care. This is the area in which we need to grow.

Chiropractic has become tagged as a pain relief specialty. In your opinion what more does it have to offer people?

People come to our practices for relief care because that is how chiropractors have educated them. Now they think that we only provide relief for low-back pain, neck pain, and headaches.

When patients come in thinking they're going to get only relief care, chiropractors can vertically grow their practice through education. The chiropractor can educate young parents so they understand that chiropractic truly is broader and offers far more than just relief care. After being educated, these patients then have the option to practice a more wellness-oriented lifestyle.

Growing a practice vertically simply means that while one member of the family may come in for relief care, the rest of the family comes in because they understand it's not for the pain or symptoms, but rather because they really embrace this wellness lifestyle.

Chiropractic care is this lifestyle's foundation and nutrition is also a component. For many people, nutrition is a blind spot in their life because of the Western culture's emphasis on fast and processed foods.

Promoting a wellness lifestyle also means teaching people to become mindful, listen to their bodies, and to not ignore them. So, teaching mindfulness is another core component.

Yet another is the lifestyle habits involved in raising a healthy family; everything from choosing a proper baby carrier, to sport choices, and other activities for the children. The majority of young chiropractors are raising *their* own families in healthful ways to begin with, so why not take all of the great choices they're making for their children — organic foods, good sleep habits, and things that make a difference in a child's quality of life — and use them as resources for their patients?

What is the purpose of the chiropractic adjustment and how does not receiving chiropractic care impact one's life?

One of the most important things we, as chiropractors, ought never to forget is how powerful the adjustment is, and not take it for granted. It's important that chiropractors don't get too used to or mindless about the adjustment. If they do, they become technicians who just manipulate joints. So many people out there are doing manipulation, but that is **not** a chiropractic adjustment.

The more that chiropractors become artists with their adjustments, the more powerful effect those adjustments will have for their patients. Some doctors think, "Oh, I just give an adjustment." No, wait a second! Our whole life as chiropractors revolves around giving an adjustment. We must never forget the passion of delivering that adjustment.

I'm saddened when I learn of a person who doesn't receive adjustments because for my whole life I knew that when my body wasn't functioning well I'd go down the hallway, wake up my dad, and tell him I needed an adjustment. I didn't know that health came from anywhere else so I can't even imagine the concept of a life of not being adjusted.

People who aren't being adjusted are walking in the Valley of the Dark. Giving that gift of the chiropractic adjustment allows them to walk in the Valley of the Light. What we are truly doing is helping them facilitate their journey and when they make a choice to include chiropractic as a part of that, they're on their way.

People have a natural desire to be in the light — I think it's innately driven. It's instinctive, but sometimes if they have walked in the Valley of the Dark for too long, even if you gave them a flashlight they wouldn't even know how to push the on button!

What is your favorite quote and how has it impacted your life?

I have many quotes that, at different stages of my life, have had an impact, so I really don't have an answer. I keep my quotes to myself and know that they personally move me. I will mention, though, that we have a time and weather display outside the office and for the last 15 years we've placed positive quotes on it and more than 40,000 vehicles pass by daily. We often get phone calls or handwritten notes from people thanking us for a quote and telling us how it made a big difference in their lives. I am a big believer in the power of words.

How is chiropractic unique and what does it offer that other health professions do not?

The primary factor is our philosophy. What makes us unique is that with so little — just by using our hands — we can move mountains. We don't need to live a life of high-tech, like so many other health professions. From the beginning, from the first adjustment, it's a matter of just remembering our science, art, and philosophy. That is what I think sets us apart.

There will be advancements in chiropractic but we really are pretty much the originals and not much has changed. One thing about the philosophy of chiropractic is how pure it is. It's very pure in the fact that our philosophy teaches people how to live from above, down, inside, out. The chiropractic philosophy incorporates and encompasses the spirituality of life, the way D.D. and B.J. Palmer wrote about.

We're very fortunate to have had them as the discoverer and developer, respectively. Today, people who are studying quantum physics and holistic care are actually embracing our philosophy and redefining it a little bit to fit themselves.

What do you sense was the intention behind the creation of chiropractic?

I believe D.D. Palmer was an inventor. He was obviously very curious and attracted to health and the human body, which he had studied before creating chiropractic. He was a learner and was hungry for learning. I don't think that it was coincidental that he gave that first adjustment to Harvey Lillard, who was deaf and "just happened" to have a subluxation and interference to his function. I don't think it was coincidence. I think it was Divine.

B.J. Palmer, the developer of chiropractic, was a bridge builder. He had many interests and knew many people and was able to work with them. One of the things we ought to become better at today is bridge building with our community and with all other people in our lives.

Who are some of your mentors and what impact have they had on your life?

I'd have to start with my mother and father, just for the fact that they instilled in me the understanding that I can do anything. My dad has always been so powerful even though he's a man of few words. He says very little and yet I witnessed him move mountains by adjusting patients. People would come to him just because they wanted to experience the art of the adjustment. My dad taught me to value the chiropractic adjustment and to be the best adjuster.

One of my other mentors is Clarence Gonstead, an amazing adjuster who was always trying to figure out how to deliver a better adjustment. He was an extraordinary inventor, too. I appreciated that because being able to deliver a better adjustment means we can alter physiology — and the body knows what to do with that.

From an educational point of view, I have to say thank you to Joe Flesia and Guy Riekeman. I was a student when they started teaching their Renaissance Seminars and they greatly influenced me to embrace the science, art, and philosophy in a professional manner. They were extremely instrumental people in my life.

What are some things, if any, you had to give up in order to devote your life to chiropractic?

It's definitely the opposite. I really can't say that I've given up anything; it's been a wonderful choice and I haven't given up anything. Of course, there are certain points in life where I thought about other roads I could have taken, how I could have done this or that, or what if I had made that choice. But I have no regrets. It's funny because sometimes when I think that it can't get any better than this, it still does! I didn't give up anything. I just made a different choice. It was a great choice and it has been a wonderful journey.

What turns you on creatively, spiritually, or emotionally?

Finding ways to create good educational messages turns me on. I love problem solving. I find it very creative to come up with better messages via teaching workshops, PowerPoint presentations, newsletters, and figuring out how to be a better communicator.

I get excited about creating a better teaching tool. I love seeing the tools I created help other chiropractors expand their practices. That just gets me going and I feel things cannot get any better than that. Creating is probably one of the most exciting parts of my life.

As for the spiritual part of life, I am grateful to have grown up in a Christian faith that I absolutely love. I have been blessed in that it was such a great place to have grown up. I still maintain my active faith and it allows me to love others and I am very grateful to be able to express it in this manner.

Where do you see the profession 10 years from now?

When it comes to the care of children and families under chiropractic care, one of the saving graces of our profession will be the fact that there are 3,000 souls committed to going out there and providing chiropractic care for families.

This is thanks to the International Chiropractic Pediatric Association (ICPA), which I have been involved with for the last 27 years. The organization has grown to 3,000 members strong, publishes *Pathways* magazine, and has developed certification and Diplomate programs.

We are really true to our mission that every child should have the right to have an adjustment. Some out there would like to limit chiropractic care to only six adjustments, can you imagine that? I do really believe that the ICPA could be the saving grace.

What profession other than your own would you like to have attempted?

When you're 6 years old and know what you want to do with the rest of your life, it's kind of hard to say, "Oh, did I make a mistake?" My answer could be different five years from now, but I think it would have been intriguing to go into law or become either a politician or an ambassador.

Maybe part of that is from my European upbringing and the love of different cultures. I think also, since I'm so proud to be an American and admire our wonderful system, it would have been an interesting direction to have been an advocate for the people. I feel that I am an advocate for children and pregnant moms in our profession and I think I would have been an interesting advocate on a political level.

Are there any other comments you'd like to share about the wonders of chiropractic?

When chiropractors realize that the most powerful thing they can do is give the adjustment, and how powerful the adjustment is, they have a sense of confidence that some of their colleagues are lacking.

With that lack of confidence, some chiropractors don't see the miracles many of us see on a daily basis — the miracle of life, the miracle of improved quality of life, the miracle of just seeing people healthy, and the joy that comes from all that.

For my colleagues, I would like to give the hope of going back to the roots of adjusting and remind them never to give up being an educator, which is something you will do every moment of your practice life. Never forget that part of your mission is to be the best educator for your community because that's how others are going to learn about chiropractic.

Years from now when people look at your tombstone, what would you want them to read?

I don't think I need anything written on my tombstone. I lived my life and I touched the lives that I touched and that will be my living legacy. Not words on stone but the love or the actions that may have touched (hopefully) thousands of chiropractors' lives, who in turn, touched thousands of their patients' lives. My legacy won't be on a tombstone, it will be in the lives of people.

Claudia Anrig, D.C., has been in full-time practice for the past 27 years and is the founder of the first comprehensive pediatric program and community outreach, Peter Pan Potential. Through her "Generations" coaching program, she also personally mentors chiropractors who dream of growing their family wellness practice.

Dr. Anrig is the past president and currently serves on the board of the International Chiropractic Pediatric Association and is on the post-graduate faculty of Life University, Life Chiropractic College West, Northwestern Health Sciences University, and Cleveland Chiropractic Colleges — Kansas City and Los Angeles.

She received the "Chiropractor of the Year" award for 1997 from the World Chiropractic Alliance, Fellow of the International Chiropractic Association (ICA) in 1997, and Distinguished Service from the ICA in 1998. Dr. Anrig's textbook, "Pediatric Chiropractic," is the first of its kind and is the fastest-selling textbook in chiropractic history.

The difference between what we do and what we are capable of doing would suffice to solve most of the world's problems.

Gandhi

Arno Burnier

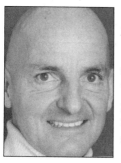

Where are you from originally and what was your childhood like?

I was born and raised in downtown Paris, about five minutes from the Eiffel Tower. I grew up in a conservative, upper-middle-class bourgeois French family with a father who was pretty much never home and a mother who had been severely wounded and had a heart of stone.

My childhood was pretty much resigned to isolation and non-validation of my being. Both of my parents were perfectionists, so there was a high demand to be perfect at all times and I was not lovable unless I was perfect.

That was very much the theme of my childhood, combined with a really tragic environment around my brother and sister. My brother made many attempts at suicide, one of which I was a witness — with the bathroom full of blood everywhere.

My sister was really a social recluse because she had been sexually violated and abused, not just one time but on a regular basis pretty much every week. After that, it was for three straight months during the summer vacation, by her step-grandfather. None of our family knew this until she was about 12 years old and, as a young woman, it all came out and she would go into violent rages against society at large and our family.

That was my childhood environment — with me at the center trying to be the mediator and conciliator.

What inspired you to get involved with chiropractic?

My early recollection is that as a young child I always had a knack for and a desire to assist people who were not feeling well and attend to wounded animals.

When I was a teenager, the only avenue I knew was medicine. When I graduated from high school, which is equivalent to two years of college in the States, I went straight into medical school for two years and then spent a year in the hospital as an extern.

I had a motorcycle crash at this time and I knew nothing about chiropractic. I had never even heard of it. A friend of my mother said I probably had a spinal injury from the accident and recommended I see a chiropractor because they were specialists from America in the spine and nerve system. That is how I was introduced to chiropractic and I met my chiropractor, Jean Belaval in Paris.

He was amazingly charismatic, passionate, and his office was filled with people who were constantly coming in and out. When he saw me as a new patient that first day, we had a powerful interaction. He listened while I told him my reason for being there and about my varied symptomatology. He pretty much connected with me with three sentences that completely blew my mind. He ignited my consciousness in that moment and I knew that, no matter what, I was going to be a chiropractor!

Where do you currently reside and how are you spending your time these days?

I reside in the mountains of Durango, Colorado at 6,500 feet. I spend my day pretty much in my home, which has beautiful views of the mountains and undisturbed scenes of nature. I ski, snowboard, hike, motorcycle, bicycle, swim, and when I am not doing those things, I am totally committed to chiropractic. I spend a lot of my time communicating with the profession, answering e-mails, supporting students in the transition from college into practice, supporting chiropractors, teaching an adjusting seminar, teaching what used to be the "Camp" and is now called The IP (The Involution Process), and another program called The XP (Expression Process). So, I am involved full-time with all of that.

How does the profession differ now from when you first became involved?

When I first became involved, my experience was with the chiropractor in France. He introduced me to other chiropractors who had studied in the States and were very passionate, dedicated, and committed. For them, chiropractic was a way of life. They were not **practicing** chiropractic, they were *being chiropractors.*

When I came to the States, I went to Sherman College in Spartanburg, South Carolina and was exposed to Drs. Thom Gelardi, Lyle W. Sherman, Earl Taylor, Don Thomas, Doug Gates, and Reggie Gold. They were part of the matrix of the college and were passionate, dedicated, and inspiring. That was my initial experience and exposure.

I graduated from chiropractic college in 1977 and moved to Pennsylvania. By the time I began practice, a large number of people were still very passionate about chiropractic. Today, I find that many students are completely lost. They graduate from chiropractic college having little to no understanding of chiropractic. They don't know what they are supposed to do, how they are supposed to practice, and what it is chiropractors do and don't do. They are lost.

The bulk of our profession is beginning to think, "This is just a business," or, at best, "This is just a profession." They practice three days a week, more to serve themselves than to serve the public.

Here and there, a sliver of the profession is still into the vocation of chiropractic, inspired, dedicated, committed, serving the public out of the goodness of their hearts, and from a humanitarian point of view. So, that is how I see the profession having differed.

What, if anything, needs to happen for the shift to take place to realign chiropractic with its truth and its principles?

The entire curriculum in all chiropractic colleges need to shift. Today, those curricula bury students in the mechanistic, medical, and fear-based model of life, which is not the chiropractic philosophy. The chiropractic philosophy is based on **trust** of life. It's a vitalistic model, a life model, and not a sickness model. So, the first thing that needs to change is the education.

Then, I think chiropractors need to be reminded they have been called to do this work. They have been called to be an instrument of healing, an instrument of the Divine to bring down and facilitate healing. They may have to get back into a better balance. As much as my generation and the generation before me may have been extreme in practicing six days a week, the new generations — which are "Me" generations — have gone the other way and I think the pendulum has to swing back to the center where chiropractors practice four or five days a week. They can have a long weekend, they can be well remunerated, but they have to remember to practice to serve the public.

How do chiropractic and performance relate?

I think there is a direct correlation. I know it has been argued many times, "Where is the research?" and "Where is the proof?" To me, the proof is in the customer satisfaction. We know that when horses, especially racehorses, get adjusted, they perform better. Racehorse owners and jockeys are willing to pay $250 to have their racehorses checked for spinal subluxations before races because they know they'll perform better. The same thing has been observed with dogs at dog shows.

If it is true for horses and dogs, which have no belief system about what chiropractic does, it is surely true for human beings! We know many athletes such as Lance Armstrong and Dan O'Brien are using or have used chiropractic to help them achieve victory and win trophies.

How does chiropractic relate to a person realizing his or her fullest human potential?

Let's look at the basics. We know that if the nerve system functions better when there is no subluxation and no interference to the pathways between the brain and body; the organs, tissues, and cells physiologically perform better.

> **Sometimes, we don't think of creativity, understanding, integration, correlation, and so on as being body functions, but they are!**

If that is true of physiology, then it is true of another physiology, which is called *life expression*. Sometimes, we don't think of creativity, understanding, integration, correlation, and so on as being body functions, but they are! They are functions of the brain and functions of the nerve system. We know that chiropractic affects the physiological function of the internal organs, tissues, and cells, and by the same token it affects the function of life, which is the way we interact with, interpret, and express life.

How does chiropractic offer people an opportunity to realize an enhanced quality of life?

People can have a higher immune function, better resistance to sickness and disease, and greater adaptation to life.

Beyond that, we frequently talk about someone healing from this illness or that illness or even from cancer. But, we seldom talk about another type of miracle: people who go through life having literally zero need for medication or over-the-counter drugs, with minimal use of medical care, perhaps only for emergency repair or a critical situation. We never talk about those people.

I stumbled onto chiropractic in 1973 and I have had very, very minimal use of over-the-counter drugs and medical care. I am 58 years old now and my only use of medical care has been strictly for severe injury and repair, not for functional disorder or illnesses.

What do you feel has happened to the chiropractic profession that may have limited it from being seen by the world in its true nature?

In the early days, we had to fight the onslaught of the medical profession, which tried to crush our profession. We had to fight a legal battle with the American Medical Association — an effort led by Dr. Clair O'Dell of Michigan, co-chair of the National Chiropractic Antitrust Committee — which came to a successful conclusion for the chiropractic profession.

Once we emerged from that, chiropractic was deeply anti-medical and that legacy stayed with us until the late '70s and early '80s. Then a new wave came in who said instead of being anti-medical, we needed to be pro-chiropractic, and a shift took place. That was something that has affected the world's perception of chiropractic.

Because we are a vitalistic profession, we cannot be validated scientifically with a mechanistic yardstick, which is what the medical profession, the establishment, and the government agencies want us to do. You simply cannot evaluate a vitalistic discipline with a mechanistic yardstick. That is another hurdle, one we are still facing.

The next hurdle we've faced is the fact that, starting in the late '60s and early '70s, chiropractic became covered by health insurance. That has completely polluted our profession, polluted our graduates, and is literally the Trojan horse that severely damaged chiropractic.

Chiropractors were no longer able to practice chiropractic. Rather, they had to start practicing in a way that was incongruent with their principles. They had to practice according to the insurance industry's standards so they could get reimbursement. That has been the great downfall of our profession.

Many chiropractors have — because of the headaches and other ramifications that come with insurance — moved into cash practice, as have many dentists and MDs who no longer want to deal with the dictatorial system imposed by insurance companies.

Secondly, the entire so-called health care system in America is completely bankrupting the country. Something will have to happen and the next logical step is going to be proactive wellness care. Chiropractic is well positioned for that. The powers that be — the insurance companies and the government — need to see the wisdom in giving people an incentive to take care of themselves while they are well rather than to wait until they are sick.

Once the government supports practitioners who educate clients about a healthy lifestyle, we will see a change. Insurance companies may even change their policies and begin to reimburse a small fee for regular adjustments because they'll see the wisdom of saving money in the long term.

Chiropractic has become tagged as a pain relief specialty. In your opinion, what more does it have to offer people?

Chiropractic has definitely assisted many people to heal from their sicknesses, injuries, illnesses, and symptoms, but it's a lot more than that. If it can allow the body to function better, which means to heal better, then it can allow the body to stay well and adapt in a better way.

I mentioned before that chiropractic allows people to have a greater quality of life. B.J. Palmer always stated that the purpose of the adjustment — regardless of what appears to be, regardless of the interpretation that the person receiving the adjustment may have — is to unite man the physical with man the spiritual.

How does that take place? Very simply, Life Force in the body is the mental impulse, is the innate force, and is spirit. So, indeed, when we clear a subluxation, we release into the body more light, which is spirit, which is essence, which is Life Force, and which is vitality.

In that sense, chiropractic facilitates a greater connection between the spiritual and the physical. Throughout my journey in chiropractic, my 20 years in practice, and the last 12 years in coaching, mentoring, consulting, and teaching, my message has been that chiropractic is about helping people with aches, pains, symptoms, and disease, but it is **primarily** a lot more than that!

What is the purpose of the chiropractic adjustment and how does not receiving chiropractic care impact one's life?

The purpose of the adjustment is clearly to free the imprisoned mental impulse that has been blocked by what is basically a rheostat on the nerve system caused by subluxation. That to me is what the adjustment is about. The trickle-down effects and the byproducts are numerous and almost unforeseeable. One cannot know what will happen in a person's body after receiving an adjustment.

On the other hand, **not** receiving chiropractic care is like not receiving dental care. If you go to third world countries where people do not receive dental care, you see the devastating effect that it has not only on the esthetics of the mouth and smile, but also digestion, assimilation, etc., because they can no longer chew and eat food properly.

To me, it is in the same order. People who do not receive chiropractic care don't even know what they are missing but it has a very tangible, potent affect on them. Most do not live healthy lives. They're chronically ill, plagued with sickness and disease, and the overall cost to society is enormous.

What is your favorite quote and how has it impacted your life?

My favorite quote is from Gandhi, "What is possible for one is possible for all." I love that quote because it really dispels excuses such as "I can't do that" or "It won't happen to me" or "I can't learn that." It puts people face-to-face with what is possible if they are willing to commit, train, and eventually succeed as a result of that commitment and training. I think it is a very uplifting and encouraging quote that dispels passivity and victim behavior.

What do you sense was the intention behind the creation of chiropractic?

I think the intention was far beyond what D.D. and B.J. Palmer (founder and developer, respectively) may have even thought it was. To me, chiropractic came as an instrument of evolution to facilitate the process of enlightenment. It came at a time that was appropriate so that it could take roots among the end of the mechanistic model of life, and was timed so that chiropractic would be a more mature profession as we move into The New Era, The Age of Aquarius, The Age of Enlightenment, and the vitalistic model of life.

I think it really has nothing to do with D.D. and B.J. Palmer. It's just that the forces of the universe dropped chiropractic on the planet because a great need was emerging to facilitate enlightenment in humanity. As there is a quickening of the vibration on the planet, people's nerve systems need to be clear and opened up so they can receive higher frequency and higher vibration.

Who are some of your mentors and what impact have they had on your life?

Clearly Christ and his message of love one another, and that love is really the message. When I say Christ, I am very clear that it is not Christ from the way that religion has seen Christ. Rather, Christ from the spiritual message of Christ.

That, to me, has been a driving force: living by example. For years, there were quotes about how the messenger and the message do not have to match, and not to confuse the messenger with the message.

I think Christ clearly stated that the messenger is the message and the message is the messenger. Live by example. So, Christ is one of my mentors and Gandhi is another. Martin Luther King and John F. Kennedy are as well. Kennedy not necessarily by his behavior but by the way that he inspired the country. I especially enjoy his quote, "Ask not what your country can do for you, ask what you can do for your country."

Chiropractors frequently ask me, "What am I going to gain by coming to this seminar?" and I answer them that I cannot tell them what they're going to gain because that is an unknown — it's going to be up to them. What I ask them in return is, "What are you willing to contribute by coming to this seminar?"

If we flip the coin around and ask "What can I give ... What can I give to others ... What can I contribute to others?" rather than "What's in it for me?" we would have a very different world.

Those are my mentors — and obviously B.J. Palmer!

What are some things, if any, that you have had to give up in order to devote your life to chiropractic?

I gave up a lot of my own life. I gave up a lot of free time, vacation, and play time. I sacrificed time that I could have had with my children when they grew up, even though now that they're 23 and 25 I see my choices neither damaged nor impaired my relationship with them in any way.

I think the fact that my wife and I lived by example was an amazing inspiration for them and as a result they felt that they acquired an entire life education symbiotically. I did sacrifice a lot for chiropractic and so did my wife.

CSR: What turns you on creatively, spiritually, or emotionally?

What turns me on creatively is being in nature and reading an inspiring book on healing, spirituality, or well-being. That really inspires me creatively. Spiritually, I think I was inspired from within very early on in my life. B.J. Palmer and the chiropractic philosophy was a large piece of the exploration that still fuels the fire in my life today.

My connection with a spiritual guru from India in the early '80s, Guru Maya, has been a great inspiration to my spiritual life. I had only a quick and brief encounter with that person but from that moment forward my spiritual life became rich and I was committed to it.

Physically, I am self-motivated to exercise daily and I almost never miss a full hour of exercise each morning, along with my meditation.

That has been inspired by the chiropractic lifestyle that was "injected" into me while at Sherman College of Straight Chiropractic.

A deep connection with others turns me on emotionally, especially during the training camps we do, where we share a very deep connection and my heart completely opens up. I am very inspired by that emotionally. Obviously, my connection with my children and my wife has been a great inspiration to my emotional life as well as the recent addition of a grandchild.

Where do you see the profession 10 years from now?

My great hope is that the work that we have done over the last 12 years with Masterpiece Training Camp, whose function, vision, and purpose was to "Seed the future leadership of the profession" will have an impact. Also, I trust that Guy Riekeman being at Life University, along with a vitalistic vision, will have a great impact.

Many other wonderfully principled, committed, dedicated, and vitalistic chiropractors will all have an impact as well. They will combine with what I believe are the converging forces of life towards vitalistic and proactive health, wellness, and a healing model of life.

The combination of all of those factors gives me my great hope and vision that the profession will return to simplicity and truth with a refined delivery of the adjustment and that doctors will begin to understand that being a chiropractor is not just to adjust people.

Chiropractic is a philosophy, a science, and an art, which means that it is the adjustment, the teaching of the life principle of chiropractic, and the restoration of trust in the innate wisdom of the body through the science of innate and the science of chiropractic. So, that is my great hope and vision for the profession.

What profession other than your own would you like to have attempted?

There is no other profession I can think of that would have provided the joy, the fulfillment, and the inspiration I've gained through chiropractic, along with the gift of being able to deliver it almost anywhere and anyplace.

Are there any other comments you'd like to share about the wonders of chiropractic?

I'm always astonished by how little is needed for an adjustment on babies and children and how incredibly they respond physiologically. My greatest miracles in practice — some of them have been truly life-saving, a matter of life or death — were with babies. The parents knew very clearly that if those babies had not been adjusted, they would have died. Their medical situation was very complex and documented from some of the best children's hospitals in Pennsylvania. Then came the chiropractic adjustment and their entire physiology shifted and that child lived. So, that to me has always been the bewildering factor about chiropractic.

Years from now when people look at your tombstone, what would you want them to read?

I am clear that my legacy has been, "This man inspired us by the way he lived."

A 1977 graduate of Sherman College of Chiropractic, Paris-born **Arno Burnier, D.C.,** practiced in Pennsylvania for nearly two decades, going on to become an international guest lecturer and a team speaker at many chiropractic and health conferences and events. He was named one of America's 27 best doctors of chiropractic out of a pool of 65,000 by *Self Magazine* in August 1993.

The founder and conductor of Spinal Motion Palpation Seminars and MLS Adjusting Seminars, Dr. Burnier is also the creator and author of the ABC Conference (which demonstrates the connection between modern obstetrical procedures and neurospinal damages) and the founder and director of Master-Piece Training Camp (a six-day training camp in the philosophy, science, and art of chiropractic). Author/producer of the video, "Children & Chiropractic," he has appeared on radio and television talk shows and written numerous articles on chiropractic, health and healing, and wellness.

Dr. Burnier serves on the faculty and board of trustees of the International Chiropractic Pediatric Association.

Pasquale Cerasoli

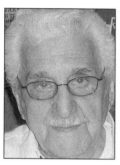

How old are you?

I am 97-plus years of age. And don't forget the plus. It's important!

Where are you from originally and what was your childhood like?

I am from South Brooklyn, New York, and I still live there. I was born two blocks from where we sit and my mother was born down the block. These are my roots, right here. When I was 3 years old, I was vaccinated for polio and developed post-vaccine encephalitis from the vaccine. I was ill so long. You can see that right from the start medicine failed me. For three months, doctors said I wouldn't live. Well, I made it but I was always sick and we tried everything. Finally, many years later, someone told me about chiropractic and I got well through chiropractic. You must realize that medicine did not work and when someone introduced me to chiropractic, something clicked inside of me, and I knew that was the way.

What inspired you to get involved with chiropractic?

I first found out about chiropractic at 29 years of age. I would drive two hours one way, three days a week, to receive an adjustment from William H. Werner, D.C., whose office was located in Queens on Woodhaven Blvd. But it was well worth the trip and I made a vow that if he ever found a cure for what ailed me, I would spend my life making sure as many people as possible found out about it.

Chiropractic healed me and I have spent my entire life defending chiropractic and bringing it to the people. You must also understand that this wonderful man introduced me to the philosophy of chiropractic. He would tell me, "There's a YOU within YOU and THAT is the healer." He impressed this on me so much that it became part of me.

CSR: Where do you currently reside and how are you spending your time these days?

I still live in Brooklyn and I pretty much spend my time as a recluse getting information in my home. You can see all of these books here that I'm reading. I am researching words and their roots. Words have much meaning and that meaning is misconstrued by society, as is chiropractic.

The real meaning of the origin of all words is not what people think they know. The same holds true for the real meaning and practice of chiropractic. I'm experiencing shortness of breath these days and I am forced to acclimate myself to this new place. I have been going through hell for the past couple of months now because it is harder to breathe.

> *Spiritually, all suffering and sickness is non-existent. It's only because of this current state of negativity and the lack of faith in our own power and existence that we have all this sickness, disease, and suffering.*

Spiritually, all suffering and sickness is non-existent. It's only because of this current state of negativity and the lack of faith in our own power and existence that we have all this sickness, disease, and suffering. For the spiritually inclined, you lose nothing and gain everything. When there is a spiritual shift in the consciousness of our world, you will see people have a shift towards chiropractic and what we are truly all about.

I still continue to go around and speak. This job is not going to go away quickly, so I will stay here until chiropractic gets back to where it was before it fell to the wayside. If it means that we have to change the whole structure of everything, then so be it. I view chiropractic as a train. When the curriculum started to follow a medical model, the chirotrain changed tracks. For years, the track has taken us in the wrong direction and labeled the profession as "musculoskeletal." I now believe the train has stopped and when it starts up again, will it keep heading in the wrong direction? We'll see to it that it doesn't!

I also teach postgraduate courses once a week on Thursday evening in the auditorium that used to serve as the lecture hall for my public chiropractic lectures. I teach the philosophy of chiropractic and adjusting to chiropractors but lay people like to come down and learn about chiropractic philosophy, so they sit in too. Chiropractors come from all over to these wonderful gatherings so they may stay focused and in touch with the essence of chiropractic. We call it the CELL-F Center.

CSR: How does the profession differ now from when you first became involved?

We had less schooling than students have now. We had three years. Our first two years were 12 months, and the last year was 10 months. The classes consisted of much of the same "stuff" as the students are getting today. We studied diagnosis, pathology, bacteriology (microbiology), histology, etc. But what you must consider is that all of these courses were slanted toward chiropractic. Back then, our chiropractic schools never followed the medical model the way they all do now.

Your question is hard for me to answer, but I'll answer from an emotional standpoint. We had a job to do and we didn't care what the law said because we realized we were working with a higher law and no other law could ever, ever stop us. I was fortunate because I was a G.I. and was more respected than the non-G.I.s who were put in jail. When these men and women were released from jail, they opened up their offices again in spite of what happened. They had the courage of their convictions. These chiropractors didn't go to jail because they were criminals; they went to jail because some "invested interest" was after chiropractic because it interfered with their monetary system.

Today, it's corporate and anything that is corporate comes from the Latin word "corpus." If you break the word down you get core, which is the heart and pus, which is filling the heart, and so it's not pure.

How does chiropractic offer people an enhanced quality of life?

It offers spirituality, where you have immortality. Let's get back to our state of chiropractic on the outside. Today, the corporate people produce a problem and you want to fix the problem. Chiropractic today is not what it should be. You have the Council on Chiropractic Education (CCE), which doesn't understand any more about chiropractic — even in the old way — than some of our lay people. It's a corporate organization now. Who the hell are these people to boss me around? Who the hell are all the corporate people to boss me around?

What do you feel has happened to the chiropractic profession that may have limited it from being seen by the world in its true nature?

One issue was when chiropractic was forced into state licensure. At that time, G.I.s were respected and this is why we were overlooked when it came down to being arrested. I believe chiropractic got its license because when the G.I.s were coming to New York to practice, the state couldn't put us in jail so they gave us a license. So, New York was the first state to be licensed. It was the kind of license that shackled the profession because it demanded (and still demands) that we study in-depth courses that follow a medical model. What's bad about this is that the depth of study has taken us away from chiropractic and put us virtually in the field of medicine. This is my argument.

We must recognize that the time will come when chiropractic will come back. Behind this plan, there is something great, some designer who designed these events this way, and we're coming back. As I've always said, I don't go away that easily!

Another issue right now is that I don't know if the perception of chiropractic by the public is as good as when I was in practice without a license. You see, we educated the public. I'm not saying that certain chiropractors don't, but the majority don't educate. I personally think they're sitting on some sort of a green grass pasture and are reaping the benefits of insurance. They are forgetting that they have a calling to assist people so they can stay in the best state of health possible. This is not a business venture. This is a higher calling, one that will ultimately see the transformation of society. I'm happy to say that in my last year of travels, I've seen more and more public lay meetings and organizations formed, so I think we're getting chiropractic back. I think the current population of chiropractors want to know and want to serve humanity.

The younger chiropractors today have a different sense of value than a decade ago. Today, they are more "spiritual" and need guidance on the correct track from someone who was there. This is why I do what I do. We should recognize that today is not yesterday and we shouldn't stop advancing just because someone said this or that years ago. We must advance and just as each past generation blossomed like a flower, so should this one — with newer and fresher petals.

A final issue is what insurance reimbursement has done to the profession. It has hurt and controlled chiropractic since it was granted. You end up no longer working for the patient, you work for the money. It has gotten to the point where chiropractors have five or six offices and associates working for them, while they're out on the golf course collecting the corporate insurance money. That type of chiropractor doesn't work for the patient or chiropractic. The simplicity of it is that all you need is a heart in its center, a chiropractic adjusting table, your hands, and seats for them to sit down on and wait for you.

What keeps the chiropractic profession splintered, divided, and separated today?

It's like a grapevine where you see the big bunch there, then it has a twig, another little bunch, and another little bunch, and these are all the various groups and associations. Each one starts to fight each other and they need to understand that this is not the way it should be. Chiropractic in its truth and essence can bring us all together as one.

Chiropractic in its truth and essence can bring us all together as one.

We have to start on a very simple path, the way we once did. There was once a bunch of grapes in the profession that used to yell, "Innate, Innate, Innate," and they did a very good job. Later on, when the corporate influence came in, they were afraid of that and didn't want it anymore. Fear is what motivates the corporate entities in any profession. Chiropractic has become extremely limited today, in accordance with the CCE. They say you can't do this and you can't do that. Who the hell are you to tell me what I can and cannot do?

CSR: How is the shift in chiropractic going to take place from a corporate to a spiritual setting you are talking about?

A handful of people are all that are needed to make the shift. CELL-F Center has plenty of people already. In chiropractic, we look at the neural system (not the nervous system, because no one likes to be nervous). The neural system is going to be a new system and more complicated than it is now, although it will not be a house divided. If you look at the so-called nervous system today, you will see that the parasympathetic system is a house divided. You have the cranial and you have the sacral, which is a house divided. How the hell can we have internal affairs working as they should when we are a house divided inside ourselves? We have to undergo our metamorphosis.

What is the purpose of the chiropractic adjustment and how does not receiving chiropractic care impact one's life?

As a chiropractic servant, I don't adjust people. All I do is serve them and they adjust themselves. This is another misconception, that the chiropractor adjusts people. That's B.S. The chiropractor simply sends in a force and they take that force and internally turn it into their own power to adjust themselves. Chiropractors who tell you that we can straighten out spines and all of that are forcing the issue and could hurt people. This is why we are so splintered in chiropractic. There are too many voices, opinions, and interpretations of what chiropractic is.

There is truly only one voice, no opinions, or interpretation. When delivering the thrust to the person on the table, it must be done at a specific time and with honor for who is on that table.

What is meant by the vertebral subluxation?

A subluxation can have a couple of meanings. One is sub, where there is not enough light. The next time it could mean even something better: sub-luxation which means the light above shining upon the nation below. Which one do you want? You have to be careful about new stuff you are bringing in to replace the old. We are not bringing in anything from the outside now. We are bringing in things from the inside.

The chiropractic profession has been off center for some time. With all the corporate people out there, and all their so-called advanced technology with computers, they are nothing more than off center. People have to go someplace to get their information. You have to be very careful what you are reading. Investigate words, know the true meaning of things, and dig deeper to get to know and see things in their true light.

There is a big problem with the identity of the profession and we are trying to fix it from the outside but it cannot be done that way. Somebody asked me, "What can you do for cancer?" I told them they were asking the wrong question. What can I do to *prevent* cancer is more useful because I don't want to have cancer and then try to fix it.

What impression did B.J. Palmer, the developer of chiropractic, make on you?

He once said, "Let the God above flow through your INNATE below." When he mentioned that, do you think that he saw something greater than INNATE in the body? Ask yourselves that! Philosophy is ever-growing, it just doesn't stop. The founders left us a model to work with, not a tub of polish and an old cloth to rub it repeatedly so it stays shiny. Rather, we must get our hands dirty and add to the model. We aren't meant to follow these people into their graves. Adding to chiropractic doesn't change it; it just makes it easier to understand.

CSR: If you could put a number on how many adjustments you delivered in almost 40 years of practice, how many would it be?

1,093,000.

Can you share with us some memorable changes experienced by some of your patients?

One I can share is about a fellow I grew up with who was an undertaker. When I opened up my little office in Brooklyn, he came to see me. He told me he had headaches caused by an inoperable tumor. When he asked if I could give him relief, I told him, "The only thing I can do is adjust you and if you're meant to get well, if your body will heal itself, then so be it."

I made it very clear to all of my patients that I'm not a healer — they are the healers. After three or four months, the man had no more headaches. He went back to the M.D.s and got X-rays. Sure enough, the tumor was gone. I made sure to warn him not to tell the M.D.s that he went to a chiropractor, because in those days I was an outlaw. He couldn't resist, so as he was leaving the M.D.'s office, he stuck his head back in the door and yelled, "By the way, I went to a chiropractor." This man died 12 years ago with no tumor.

In 1940, when you decided to become a chiropractor, what was your mission?

My mission was to serve sick people because I was sick all those years. When I found chiropractic, I too wanted to serve those who were suffering as I had been. In 1914, at 3 years old, I got post-vaccine encephalitis and for 17 long years, until 1930, I suffered. I wanted to get well and I was given that avenue through chiropractic. Because of this, my mission was to deliver to others the same thing that had helped me. By no means did I only focus on the sick. I also went out and told everyone about chiropractic and its benefits.

What do you sense was the intention behind the creation of chiropractic?

D.D. Palmer, in his two books, gives us information about how he received chiropractic through a spirit entity called Jim Atkinson. Who was Atkinson? He never tells us more than he was a spiritual being. As far as I can see — and it's hard to gather records from that time — D.D. was a spiritualist and belonged to spiritual community church. When he got this information, he went to his spiritual guide and he was told that his discovery was going to lead to spirituality. He then came up with the slogan: "When the physical becomes spiritual."

He said that when the human mind has inspiration or wants to go forward, it will. D.D. knew and even made prophecies that chiropractic one day would empty the jails, infirmaries, and hospitals. To me, D.D. was a prophet more than an originator.

I knew people who knew D.D., and they gave me other information as well. One person in particular said D.D. was told how to give the adjustment and where to go. So, how can we ever say it was an accident? This was a gift given to us on a silver platter.

I disagree with D.D. when he says he "discovered" chiropractic. It would be like me telling you to go under a specific tree with a shovel, dig there and you'll find a treasure. If you do, you haven't discovered it. Rather, you found it with some guidance. Also, I don't believe chiropractic has been "founded" yet because we are all "founding" it until we reach rock-bottom. Once we get to the rock-bottom and chiropractic can really express itself in its true light, what we're doing today will be "pip-squeaks" compared to what will really happen. When this day arrives, the blind will see, the lame will walk, and so forth and so on. But we cannot have it if we follow a medical model, we must stay pure.

The word "chiropractic" is from Greek and means "to do by hand." But the fact we do something by hand means nothing more than being a one-armed paper hanger! That's all we are. Actually, chiropractic is a misnomer and the name has to be changed. Not that chiropractic has to change, but the name does. Thoughts are things and every time you say something, the thought behind it comes out.

People say I'm old fashioned and I say bulls——! I am what I am. When chiropractic was given to us, he who gave it to us meant well and it was done so on purpose. But when it was given to us, we became nothing more than one-armed paper hangers, you got it? You can never get spirituality from a one-armed paper hanger.

Who are some of your mentors and what impact have they had on your life?

My spiritual teachers. They told me to continue searching, that I have to do my own work, and that they cannot do my work for me. If they work for me it does not belong to me, but if I unravel this thing, then it belongs to me and I become it.

Where do you see the profession 10 years from now?

It will be gone as we know it today, and it will become a spiritual practice. Wait until 2012 and see what happens. Chiropractic will be around and it will be different than it is today. The chiropractor will have to go on missions and heal the sick. There will be a lot of sick people around who will want to be helped. If they want to be helped, plenty will help them.

Are there any other comments you'd like to share about the wonders of chiropractic?

Chiropractic is founded on **tone**. It behooves all of us to find out just what this tone is. It is my belief that the human body is one big orchestra and each organ is an instrument that must tune itself up. But, we need a central tone someplace. Is that central tone in us lost and if it is lost, where is it? How can chiropractic help tone come back so all of these organs can be tuned to it?

When this happens, there will be no more suffering, want, illness, or tears. I'm bold enough to say that it will take the chiropractic profession to make this a reality. My spiritual brethren and friends always said to me that when you recognize what it's all about, you'll say that it is so simple and wonder why you never saw it before. We cannot look for more than what it is.

?▲

Pasquale Cerasoli, D.C., practiced seven days a week in Brooklyn, New York for 33 years, seeing well over 150 patients a day, and taking just three vacations during that time. When he began practicing in 1947, he charged $2.00 an adjustment. At his retirement, he was charging $3.00 — and children were always free. He took down his shingle in 1980 "so the young ones could have the limelight and the so-called mature people could sit back a bit."

Dr. Cerasoli remains as dedicated to chiropractic as he was in 1940 when he first discovered the profession at the age of 29. Today, he still teaches post-graduate courses once a week in the auditorium that used to serve as the lecture hall for his lay lectures.

Dr. Pat, as everyone called him, attended Eastern Chiropractic Institute, which was located in Manhattan and became a part of National College of Chiropractic.

Within each of us lies the power of our consent to health and sickness, to riches and poverty, to freedom and to slavery. It is we who control these, and not another.

Richard Bach

Gerard Clum

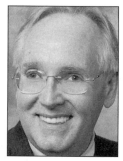

Where are you from originally and what was your childhood like?

I was born and raised in Buffalo, New York. My father was in the bakery and restaurant supply business. We had a blue collar family life and dad had his own business. My brother was the first in our family to go to college and I was the second. It was not like we came from a professional background or anything of that nature.

I had a very profound experience with chiropractic care at the age of 12. As a result of that experience, I knew I wanted to be a chiropractor. I never had any of those adolescent questions about what to do with my life — I wanted to be a chiropractor.

Frankly, the people around me found it kind of disconcerting that I was not looking at other options and wasn't considering the full range of possibilities I could choose from. I wanted to be a chiropractor. I never had any question, I never had any confusion, and I never had any pointing or leanings in any other direction. If anything, I would have enjoyed staying in the Buffalo area and getting in business with my dad. We had a great relationship and I would have liked that but it would not have been my calling.

What inspired you to get involved with chiropractic?

The experience when I was 12 years old. I developed a condition where I had lost a great deal of vision and it deteriorated to 20/800 correctible to 20/200. At that point, you are not seeing a heck of a lot. My parents were told that bilateral optic atrophy was significant and a possible precursor to multiple sclerosis. The ophthalmologist said I was either in the early stages of MS or I was dealing with a tumor at the optic chiasm.

So, at 12, I started a sequence of diagnostics. MRIs did not exist at the time and neither did CT scans or other things of that nature. I went through spinal taps, plain film radiography, and a procedure called a pneumoencephalogram. Today, young radiologists wouldn't even know what that is. They put you into a fetal position in a chair, anesthetize you, drain the cerebral spinal fluid, inject air into the ventricles (into the space) so there's a contrast between the air density in the ventricles and the water density in the brain and you're able to get an image.

The downside was that I woke up two days later convinced my brain had been sucked through the floor of my skull. That was the testing I had and the condition was determined to be idiopathic and in all likelihood progressive. I didn't have much of a future as far as eyesight was concerned.

My dad had been seeing a chiropractor — Dr. Cassan — in southern Ontario (we lived in Buffalo and had a summer home in Canada). We had been in Cleveland for a couple of weeks for more testing, and when we returned, Dr. Cassan asked my dad why he'd missed a couple of appointments.

We were the last patients of the evening and dad started to explain my condition. This fellow took out a copy of "Gray's Anatomy," Guyton's physiology text, and another pathology book. My dad was a smart man but had only a 10th grade education; he knew his business and knew it well, but he was intimidated by educated people.

When Dr. Cassan started to dissect what bilateral optic atrophy progressive vs. idiopathic meant, I remember watching the fear and suffering drain from my dad's face. For the first time, the words had meaning and he could get his hands around what they meant. I had no more or less of a problem at that point but he understood things differently at that moment.

Over the years, I've thought about all of the things chiropractic has given me, but for a young kid to watch his dad be relieved of that kind of burden, I could be in tears right now.

It was quite an experience and at the end of that conversation Dr. Cassan said to my dad, "You know Don, I don't know if I can help the boy but I guarantee I wouldn't hurt him, and I would love the chance to try." I got my first adjustment that night. Two months later, we went back to the ophthalmologist and he proclaimed that a miracle had taken place — until he heard there was a chiropractor involved and then the miracle went out the window.

At that point, my vision was now correctible from 20/200 to 20/90 and it continued to improve over the years. I went to school on the vocational rehab program because of my eyesight, but my eyesight improved and eventually I qualified for a driver's license at 20/60. I have been getting on with my life ever since.

So, that was where it all started. Aside from the adjustments and the results I had, it was the character and quality of Dr. Cassan that really gave me my first introduction to chiropractic. As a 12-year-old kid, I was conflicted because I wanted to be like my dad but I also wanted to be like this guy. That was really an important moment for me.

Where do you currently reside and how are you spending your time these days?

Well, I'm gainfully employed! My wife Cathy and I live in San Leandro, California, which is in the east San Francisco Bay area and for the last 28 years I've been president of Life Chiropractic College West. Prior to that, I was on the faculty of Life University (then Life Chiropractic College) in Marietta, Georgia. In fact, I was one of the first three faculty members when Life University — then Life Chiropractic College — opened.

There was Charlie Kalb, who now practices up in North Georgia, and a fellow by the name of Ron Watkins who has since passed away. We were the faculty at that time. Dr. Sid Williams was the president and the boss and we were the worker bees. So, I go way back in that environment.

Aside from my involvement with Life West, I've also served for the past 20 years as a member of the board of directors of the World Federation of Chiropractic. This current year, I'm immediate past president and for the two years before that I was president.

I've been through all of the chairs of the Association of Chiropractic Colleges. I've been an officer on the Council on Chiropractic Education (CCE), spent 20 years on the board of the International Chiropractors Association and one term as its vice president. I've had a lot of involvement and have been very fortunate over the years.

How does the profession differ now from when you first became involved?

The early 1970s was the time of the introduction of chiropractic into Medicare and when the CCE was in the process of being recognized by the secretary of education. Yet, other than Veterans benefits for persons who had been in the military, there was no aid to go to chiropractic college.

Chiropractic college circumstances were meager at best but, although I didn't realize it then, I now understand they did a good job with what they had to work with at that time.

The early '70s was an era when licensure was not universal in the United States. Mississippi and Louisiana had not come on board yet. We had no student loans. We had no accreditation. Inclusion in insurance programs was very sporadic and had little consistency. As a result, people who chose to be chiropractors had a conviction and a personal interest that exceeded any career potential.

I don't want to say they didn't have career potential, they did. But they were there because of some experience they had, or some experience a family member had. Something that was deeply personal and moving brought those people into the profession.

Today, the career value of chiropractic is there... but a good many people became chiropractors not so much because they wanted to do what my chiropractor first did for me, but they wanted to live in a house like he lived in or drive a car like he drove.

In 1970, there were 12,000 chiropractors in the U.S. In 2009, we're talking 70,000. A six-fold increase in essentially one long generation of chiropractors is a phenomenal growth curve.

Today, the career value of chiropractic is there — and that's not a bad thing — but a good many people became chiropractors not so much because they wanted to do what my chiropractor first did for me, but they wanted to live in a house like he lived in or drive a car like he drove. Those are fine motivations but it changed the tone of things and it changed the emphasis away from a passion of, about, and for chiropractic. That may still be there, but there's a stronger business perspective on chiropractic now. Again, there's nothing wrong with that but it's an important difference.

The other important difference is that all those things I talked about not being there in 1970 are here in 2009. Accreditation, student loans, integration into the system, chiropractors working in the military — they're all facts of life now. And there are all sorts of other things that just weren't there back then but are here now.

Each comes at a cost and changes the landscape just a little bit. Time will tell whether the cost is worth the return. But those things have all changed.

How do chiropractic and performance relate?

Chiropractic is about function and whether you're thinking about it in terms of neurological function or motor capacity or balance capacity or some other measure, everything that a chiropractic adjustment is about and is for is performance.

Human performance at some level and the performance of the human organism are essential and central to what we do, whether that performance is to heal faster, sleep better, be more physically fit and active, run a faster mile or whatever the case may be.

How does chiropractic relate to a person realizing his or her fullest human potential?

That's a leap we make as chiropractors and one we seem to make very smoothly and logically, yet it's one the public has a problem trying to absorb. People can appreciate the fact that they may be in pain on any given day and then they get an adjustment and they're out of pain. They don't quite make that jump as to the quality of life as a human being ... they are simply out of pain.

We, as chiropractors, get frustrated because people don't see the greater good of what we do but we have to go back to the perspective that a patient is a laboratory of one. The fact that you may see the impact of chiropractic 50, 100, or 200 times a day with different patients gives you a totally different perspective on and appreciation for it. But the reality is that patients see it once: when they get off that table and get back on it.

We want them to absorb our enthusiasm for chiropractic and our appreciation of the breadth and scope of the impact of what we do dramatically and quickly. But it doesn't work that way. People do not absorb life-altering things of any kind — good, bad, or indifferent — like that. It takes time and people have to process what we are providing them.

In the long run, we need to keep singing that song and keep up with that talk but we also need to bring the measures and examples down to meaningful terms rather than keep them at too high a level. We need to make it meaningful for Charlie and Mary patient on Wednesday, then again on Friday, and next Monday, so they can begin to get the accumulation of the effect of what we do. They can come to those "aha" moments and realize they truly have been feeling better since they've been seeing a chiropractor. They can come to realize their kids don't seem to get the colds they used to, and they begin to wonder about that phenomenon.

We have to meet them where they are and bring them along slowly and realize they see a fraction of what we see and therefore their response is a fraction of ours.

What do you feel has happened to the chiropractic profession that may have limited it from being seen by the world in its true nature?

It's hard to talk in those terms because in the heat of the battle and at any given moment in time you must work with what you've got. In the early '70s the profession was presented with musculoskeletal low back pain as a great need on the part of the population. It still is for that matter.

We ended up moving in that direction and lost a great deal of focus relative to neurological implications because we didn't have the evidence for it.

We went about researching low back pain because it seemed to be pretty obvious that lots of people were seeing chiropractors for that. We started emphasizing and accumulating evidence directed at the pain, disability, and worker's comp models because that's where the dollars were. Tens of millions — if not billions — were being spent in those areas and people were interested in ways to eliminate musculoskeletal and low back pain.

We ended up moving in that direction and lost a great deal of focus relative to neurological implications because we didn't have the evidence for it. On one side were the people who were dealing with an evidence-oriented world and spoke a lot about what we **did** have evidence for. Then, there were the people on the other side who were dealing with an experiential world in which they were seeing all kinds of neurological changes. Those two worlds did not connect. They did not talk to one another. The ones in the evidence world looked at the practitioner world and dismissed it as anecdotal. That caused those in the practitioner world to say, "Screw you, this is my world and I'm seeing people's lives change, so you can do all of the studies you want but I'm not interested."

We wound up having a fight between these two perspectives that is understandable but not necessary. The movement away from performance issues and into pain issues cost us in the long run. While we were consumed with that, physical therapy, osteopathy, and physical medicine were looking in other directions. We proved our case relative to the low back. We put good solid evidence on the table and then everybody else ran with our evidence. Well, we need to learn how to run with their evidence to make our case as well.

Chiropractic has become tagged as a pain relief specialty. What more does it have to offer?

I don't know that we've been tagged as pain relief, but as musculoskeletal. If we can expand musculoskeletal into neuromusculoskeletal in its full implications, it's a totally different ballgame. It gives us the potential to talk about how an upper cervical adjustment or a diversified adjustment can affect a 12-year-old kid's eyesight in a little town on Lake Erie in southern Ontario.

How does that work and what's the mechanism? For years, before we had any degree of acceptance, who the heck cared about the mechanism? Then we got a degree of acceptance and now we need to explain the mechanism.

We took the position that we can't talk about chiropractic effects until we can explain them, and this created a type of schizophrenia for the chiropractor. We were looking at measures that had clinical utility to a certain level but they were relatively meaningless to a patient. An insurance company or evaluator might like to see those measures but they had no meaning to the patient. We need to make what we do meaningful to patients.

What is the purpose of the chiropractic adjustment and how does not receiving a chiropractic adjustment impact one's life?

On a conceptual level in chiropractic, the adjustment addresses an abnormal situation and lets the body do what it wants after that.

In the pragmatic world, you can look at the purpose of an adjustment as restoring joint mobility, restoring normal kinesiopathological function, or restoring normal neurophysiology.

The bottom line is that you are allowing the body to normalize and allowing it to have a greater appreciation for its circumstances and a greater ability to integrate and relate to those circumstances.

That's the deal with the adjustment. In terms of what happens when people don't get adjusted, I think of my own situation. It's not hard for me to appreciate the fact that had I not crossed paths with that chiropractor, I could very well be blind today and my life would be radically different. Who knows? It could have been better. That's hard for me to imagine, but it could have been and I'll entertain that possibility.

But the reality is, it would be different and if I had not gotten that first adjustment and the ensuing ones, we certainly would not be sitting here talking. I would not have met my wife, nor have the career I have, nor have the children I have. The implications are endless. I never would have met someone like Dr. Sid Williams. I never would have met all sorts of people in our circle. So how do you measure the effect of withholding an adjustment?

What is your favorite quote and how has it impacted your life?

I have two quotes that come from Dr. Phil (McGraw) and they are real simple. The first is, "How's that working for ya?" The other is, "What the hell were you thinking?"

I think about the things that come across my desk, the students I deal with, the doctors who are in practice and have a problem here or there. Those two questions cover about 80 to 90 percent of what comes across my path! Sooner or later, it's a matter of, "Okay, are you going to stop and look at that and realize that's pretty stupid?" Or, "What were you thinking, pal?"

I'm sure these quotes don't sound very academic or inspirational in the larger context, but at the moment they work for me!

How is chiropractic unique and what does it offer that other health professions do not?

You know, in my earlier years in chiropractic I used to think that uniqueness was gigantic. I don't think that anymore. Many disciplines today speak about the ebb and flow of human spirit, whether they speak in terms of prana, chi, meridian flow ... or whatever. A lot of people talk our language relative to that and what I perceived as being unique and unusual in contrast to medicine is not all that unique in the marketplace. What is unique is how we bring that thinking together with the delivery of the adjustment and the significance of the adjustment as a means to alter the manifestation of flow within an individual.

As a profession, we have undervalued the adjustment. Society as a whole had a deprecating attitude toward us and therefore assumed that what we do couldn't have great value or complexity, that other people could master it quickly as well.

If you've been in chiropractic more than a month, you know that is pretty crazy. But if you're looking at it from the outside — with little respect for the discipline of the work — it's easy to disregard.

We do a lot of things that undermine the value of the adjustment. I often talk about how, as a young man, I learned to play racquetball.

I was not very good mind you, but I got the message: you hit the ball off the wall, it bounced behind the line, you stepped out of the way, and someone else hit the ball, which bounced off the wall and behind the line.

It was not a very complex game to me until I got into that box with someone who set the ball a half inch off the floor and a quarter inch behind the line at a hundred miles per hour. It was the same game ... but it was a totally different game as well.

On any given freshman orientation day, I can take the class down the hall and in 20 minutes they can move a bone, but that doesn't make them chiropractors. In that same 20 minutes, I can give them a Swiss Army Knife and a bit of Xylocaine, make an incision and they'll probably do a halfway decent job of stitching it back up. That doesn't make them surgeons.

This is way more complex than it appears! If you watch Tiger Woods play golf but have never played golf yourself, you might wonder what's the big deal? When you watch great chiropractors, it's the same way. They make it look simple, they make it look easy, they make it look effortless, and they almost make it look thoughtless.

The problem is, we never filled the gap between how easy it *looks* and the reality when people entered the game. We have undervalued what we do and we have not come up with strategies to increase the value to the public. In many ways we have followed strategies that minimize the value.

We have undervalued what we do and we have not come up with strategies to increase the value to the public. In many ways we have followed strategies that minimize the value.

What do you sense was the intention behind the creation of chiropractic?

Quite honestly, I think it was far more serendipitous then people want to think it was. Over the years, I've been involved in different meetings and circumstances and know how a situation progressed from point A to point B. Afterwards, I'd listen to various interpretations of what happened, about all these nuances and drama and stuff. Well, you know this guy left his briefcase in his room and we did it this way and there was no drama. People look at events and create all this complexity about it. If someone turned his head to the left to sneeze it supposedly meant something different than when he turned it to the right. All of this craziness we bring into it!

I think D.D. Palmer experienced something, found it fascinating, and tried to repeat it. Out of that came what we know today as chiropractic. Historically, it wasn't that unique. What was unique was the link between that procedure and the effect on the human, and then the refinement of that procedure out of a folk environment into a professional environment.

Spinal manipulation and spinal therapy of some kind go back to antiquity. All those people had spines and they had been dealing with low back and neck pain and all sorts of musculoskeletal problems. When D.D. and B.J. came along, it was the first time anyone tried to organize that body of thought and transform it into a real professional environment. That's really the significance of what went on there. I don't have these visions of God coming off Mt. Ararat to find D.D. and give him this on tablets, you know?

> **What was unique was the link between that procedure and the effect on the human, and then the refinement of that procedure out of a folk environment into a professional environment.**

Who are some of your mentors and what impact have they had on your life?

Dr. Cameron Cassan, the fellow who gave me my first adjustment, and set me on the path to become a chiropractor. I wanted to be like him. He was a wonderful guy, very caring, and loving. People appreciated the great warmth about him and he had great technical skills. He was just one of those masters who made it look easy. Aside from being a good technical chiropractor and knowledgeable fellow, he was a good man and I wanted to be that too.

My dad was the same way, a good man. He didn't really know and understand much about chiropractic other than the fact that when he got adjustments, he felt better and when he didn't get the adjustments he did not feel as good. It was a simple equation for him.

Clearly, one of my most important teachers in chiropractic was Dr. Sid Williams. I met Sid when I was 16 years old, when Dr. Cassan took me to a Dynamic Essentials meeting and I was fascinated by the guy. I didn't understand a word he said because he talked a mile a minute but I was just fascinated by him.

I later learned the value of what he was teaching and the vision he had for chiropractic for humanity, which exceeded anything that chiropractic could do by itself. I bought what he had to say hook, line, and sinker. To this day, the concept of Lasting Purpose is central to my activity and it's how I try and live my life.

What are some things, if any, you have had to give up in order to devote your life to chiropractic?

Most of my adult life I have had problems with rheumatoid arthritis. Most rheumatoid sufferers have the effects at the small joints of the hands and feet. With me, it's the big joints: knees, elbows, and that kind of thing. Full extension of my elbow, as an example, is quite limited. I started out wanting to be in practice. Still single, I taught at Palmer shortly after I graduated while I tried to figure out where I wanted to go and what I wanted to do. I got married a year later and Life College opened and I was offered the faculty position but I had every intention of practicing.

Dr. Charlie Kalb taught there and we thought we'd teach for a couple of years and they'd bring in other folks who knew what they were doing and then we'd go into practice and be done with it. I never had any respect for college administrators. I thought they weren't good chiropractors and that's why they were doing what they were doing. It's probably quite karmic that I should be where I am today — it's my payback for that! I probably have some students on my campus making that same judgment about me.

When I think about it, did I give up practice? Well, with my arthritis problems, I wouldn't have stayed in practice, so I don't know that I've had to give up anything. I've received so many things — from my health to my personal circumstances to the ability to contribute to other people's lives. I've had great experiences all over the globe. If I had taken a different path, I think it's a safe bet that I would have made more money. College presidents aren't paupers, but they're certainly not rolling in dough. At least this one isn't. But if you asked me to trade the money for where I am at today, I wouldn't trade. It would be crazy.

What turns you on creatively, spiritually, and emotionally?

Creatively, I'd like to think I'm a pretty good teacher and I love the challenge of taking a complex subject and bringing it down to something that relates to this morning's newspaper headlines. That way, people can understand the contextual nature of things in terms they can appreciate.

Anybody can rattle off information and have students turn around and vomit it back at them. The best teachers are those who give the best examples, metaphors, and models. I think I'm pretty good at that and I like to do that. I find great joy in watching people in the audience have an "aha" moment. I'll see a look in their eyes or a nod of their head that tells me they're thinking, "Oh, I get it now." That's really pretty cool and I really like that.

I love the idea of being able to contribute to the next generation or generations of chiropractors to come, in payment for what I have been given and the experiences I've had. I could never pay it forward enough.

In terms of morally and spiritually, I don't like people being unfair, that pisses me off. Whether we're talking about a teacher in the classroom or someone in Afghanistan, or anything in between. I have my Don Quixote moments where I tilt at the windmill and want to bring back chivalry but I'm motivated by those kinds of inequities and the effect they have on people.

I'm also cognizant that my life is radically different from life for the majority of people on this planet today or who have ever been on this planet. It's phenomenal to think of the good fortune we have and I try not to lose sight of that. I think of all the places on this planet that I could have been born and how my life would be nowhere near what it is today. I think to myself, "Holy mackerel, how did that happen?" The "why me?" part of it. Why am I not some goat herder in the Sudan or whatever? That has fascinated me for a long time.

Where do you see the profession 10 years from now?

I see the profession doing well and the ideas, concepts, and goals we have talked about as a discipline being widely accepted. I also see the profession being unable to accept the fact that we're now moving with the mainstream. Because we went against the stream for so long, it's become part of our genetic code to go against the stream.

I think we're going to see a great deal of refinement about what we do. We're going to look back and realize that the chiropractic I grew up on and the chiropractic I practiced and taught were pretty primitive. We'll have better ways of doing things, more efficient ways, and better measures, and we will know a lot more about when a person needs an adjustment or when they do not. We won't rely totally on intuition and sense. Not that those will ever be out of the deal, but we will see the emphasis change. Our biggest challenge will be to realize that the world has awakened to what we said and we are, in a sense, going to be like the dog that caught the car — now what the hell do I do with it?

What profession other than your own would you liked to have attempted?

I made my decision to be a chiropractor at 12. I suppose I could see myself hustling in the food business as my dad did, simply because I had some experience with it. As I look at other disciplines, the one area I think I could enjoy would be emergency medicine. The potential to make, in an instant, an impact on a person's life in a profound way when they are very vulnerable would be rewarding. I don't know any other areas of medicine I would find particularly attractive but that one has some pull.

Are there any other comments you'd like to share about the wonders of chiropractic?

Never, never, never, underestimate the value of an adjustment. The idea of undervaluing an adjustment and either not pursuing a course of care long enough or — God forbid — not pursuing a course of chiropractic care at all bothers me deeply.

Also, something Dr. Sid Williams talked about for years and years and years is so important: in our pursuit of information and technology and all kinds of things, remember that we are never going to "engineer" out the person. There is something special about the touch of another human being. I have no idea how to quantify, explain, or appreciate it, but I pray we never lose that and I pray we continue to keep a focus on that personal contact.

At each year's freshman orientation, I talk about the power of people's thoughts and their relationship to what the individuals are doing. As an example, I generally ask an attractive girl in the audience, "If you were in a bar on a Saturday night and two gentlemen came up and spoke to you and they used the exact same words, exact same mannerisms, the exact same body language, and the exact same tone of voice but one was being friendly and cordial and one was hitting on you, how long would it take you to tell the difference?"

The answer always comes back in nanoseconds. They just know. The answer I get is always, "Before they open their mouth to speak to me." Even in a bar, where there are all kinds of distractions and input coming at you, we are so acutely attuned to other people we can pick up that distinction just from the approach of the individual.

Now, take that ability into a clinical situation. I come in for your help. I'm vulnerable and needy. Do you really think your thoughts, orientation, emphasis, and attitude don't come through your hands? Don't come through a scalpel? Don't come through a prescription pad? My God, that's crazy. That's crazy! That's something in time I think we will appreciate so much more than we ever did.

Years from now when people look at your tombstone, what would you want them to read?

He was a nice guy. He was a nice man. That'll be plenty.

Gerard W. Clum, D.C., is a 1973 Palmer graduate who has been a faculty member at Palmer College of Chiropractic, a founding faculty member at Life Chiropractic College, and the first and only president of Life Chiropractic College West.

Dr. Clum has served on the board of directors or as an officer of the Association of Chiropractic Colleges, the Council on Chiropractic Education, the International Chiropractors Association (ICA), the Foundation for Chiropractic Progress, and the World Federation of Chiropractic. He is the immediate past president of the World Federation of Chiropractic.

The most senior chiropractic college administrator in the world, having served as president for more than 28 years, Dr. Clum has been recognized as "Chiropractor of the Year" by the ICA, "Man of the Year" by *Dynamic Chiropractic* and as one of the top five leaders of the chiropractic profession in a *Dynamic Chiropractic* readers' poll.

John F. Demartini

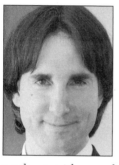

Where are you from originally and what was your childhood like?

I was born in Houston on Thanksgiving Day in 1954 with my hand and foot turned in, what they termed "pigeon foot and hand." By the time I was walking, I had to wear braces. I wore those braces until I was about 4. I wanted out of those braces and the second I got out of them I became a runner. I ran everywhere because I wanted to catch up with everybody who was able to easily walk and run.

I faced another challenge in first grade. I had some learning difficulties in addition to the initial physical problems. I was told by my first-grade teacher that I would never be able to read, write, communicate, amount to anything, or go very far in life. The only way I made it through school was by asking the smartest kids a bunch of questions. I learned how to ask quality questions to get through life.

My parents moved from Houston to Richmond, Texas to get away from the city. While I was there, I didn't have a bunch of smart kids to ask questions to and I started to fail. The main sport I excelled at was baseball, but it was infiltrated by gang members and you'd get beaten up if you struck somebody out.

I ended up dropping out of school, hanging out and living on the streets, and eventually hitchhiking to California and flying to Hawaii to be a surfer. I surfed mainly along the North Shore of Oahu and lived there as a truly dedicated surfer. I was in a surf movie, magazines, and hung out at contests.

At 17, I nearly died of strychnine poisoning and, during my recovery I met Paul C. Bragg, the inspired naturopath and longevitist. He gave an evening talk in Hawaii and inspired me to become a teacher, healer, philosopher, and to travel the world. That's when I decided I wanted to be involved in a healing profession, and be a philosopher and teacher. That's what I've been focusing on for more than 37 years.

What inspired you to get involved with chiropractic?

After meeting and learning from Paul Bragg I made an attempt to go back to school and had to overcome learning difficulties. I wanted to be involved in healing because the strychnine poisoning damaged my neuromuscular system. Because of that challenge, I studied anything and everything I could that had to do with healing.

I worked as a night watchman in a large health food store that had a huge library and I read every book there. I went to college as a pre-med student, but was never satisfied with the medical route. I never felt that we had an excess of organs or a deficiency of drugs inside our bodies.

I was looking for some form of internal and natural healing, because Paul Bragg was a naturopath. I considered going into that, but it was more limited and only a few states had recognized it as a profession.

Each summer and Christmas while I was going to school I would hitchhike somewhere and go surfing. When I was 22, I planned to go to the Hawaiian island of Kaua'i for the summer but while waiting for the plane, I got talked into going to Peru instead. Actually, I got on a plane to Miami and it was hijacked by a Cuban hijacker and we landed in Lima!

I ended up surfing at Chicama Bay and the Mira Flores beaches in Peru and while there I met the son of the governor and ended up staying at the governor's palace. The governor told me that if I was going to be in Peru, I had to go to Machu Picchu. I hitchhiked toward Chile and Arequipa, took a train ride up into the mountains to the city of Cusco, and went to Machu Picchu.

I had left my surfboard in Lima and had a backpack filled with about 20 books from the health food store! Lo and behold, one of those books was "The Chiropractic Story" by Marcus Bach.

I read that book early one morning sitting at Machu Picchu. I became inspired to tears upon realizing that the thing I'd been looking for was not naturopathy and definitely not medicine. I fell in love with the philosophy of chiropractic. Everything I'd read by the great philosophers — and everything I knew about different healing arts — all of a sudden made sense and tied together.

At that moment, at Machu Picchu, I knew I was going to be a chiropractor. I left and spent the rest of the summer hitchhiking throughout six Central American countries. I came back to the States, applied to, was accepted at, and enrolled in Texas Chiropractic College, where I finally became a licensed Dr. of Chiropractic!

Where do you currently reside and how are you spending your time these days?

Until about four years ago, I had 11 homes around the world. Now I have five and I'm very rarely at any of them. The one I most consider as "home" is *The World of ResidenSea,* a condominium ship that circumnavigates the earth. It just so happens to be down in Peru right now. I get off and on the ship and I travel pretty much 360 days a year. I'm dedicated to researching, writing, traveling, and teaching. I'm involved in helping, healing, and personal development. Last week, I was in Japan. Then I went to Milan, London, Albuquerque, Santa Fe, Dallas, and now Calgary — all in the last 10 or so days. I travel full time, speak, and reach as many millions of people as possible.

How does the profession differ now from when you first became involved?

It has had to make adaptations to the environments it has faced. When I went to chiropractic college, chiropractors were considered quacks. By the 1980s, people were calling chiropractors "unorthodox." Then it was branded as an alternative, then as complementary, and it has just gradually become mainstream.

I've watched it evolve in the last 30 years or so and there have been pains and pleasures along the way. There have been strides and setbacks. The essence of chiropractic — that the power that made the body can heal the body — is a great and grand principle that the world deserves to hear and experience. That is still there.

Obviously, there are various factions within chiropractic and various viewpoints that are usually complementary opposites that support and challenge each other. Overall, I think it is a viable profession that will continue to grow. It all depends on the visionary leaders who guide it.

If we have a leader who is a bit more fundamental and stagnant, we stagnate. Our profession vacillates between progressive leaders and those who are more subordinate to outside authorities and other healing arts. Overall, it just keeps progressing, changing, and adapting to meet the market needs.

How do chiropractic and performance relate?

Without question, when people receive chiropractic adjustments, their performance increases. I remember a lady who came to me when I was in my first year in practice. She was in her 20s and was the number one broker in Texas at the time and was even featured on the front cover of "Inc." magazine.

She came in because her neck was sore from being on the telephone in a slanted position hours every day. I suggested she get a headset and she did. I also suggested she get a bigger Rolodex so she wouldn't be cramped over, and get chiropractic adjustments before she developed further degeneration in her neck.

She started receiving adjustments. She received care for about a week. Then she disappeared. I called her but she didn't answer. Finally, about a week later, she came back in and said, "Dr. Demartini, do you think it's possible that your adjustments could be helping me perform better at work?" I told her they certainly could.

"I noticed when I was getting adjustments nearly every day, I had my biggest week," she explained. "I thought it was coincidental at first. I also noticed that when I was away from you for another week or so, it dropped down again to its average. I'd like to do an experiment. I'd like to come in here three times a week and just see if it increases my performance."

In almost every area of life, one's performance, effectiveness, and efficiency increases by having regular chiropractic care.

She did that and if I found subluxations, I would adjust her. If I didn't find any, I would leave her spine alone. During that time, she increased her business so much she considered chiropractic as one of the key elements to her ongoing success.

It wasn't only the adjustments, but also my advice, nutritional and postural suggestions, and inspiration. Chiropractic care made a huge impact on her performance.

I have many cases of people who perform better at work, are able to make love and have children, and have an improved ability to perform in school. In almost every area of life, one's performance, effectiveness, and efficiency increases by having regular chiropractic care.

How does chiropractic relate to a person realizing his or her fullest human potential?

Since ancient times and in the ancient Eastern mystical writings of the Yogis, the spine has been considered the primary axis of our existence. If the spine isn't flexible, if it's not aligned and not functioning properly, the fullest expression of our spiritual and physical existence is not maximized.

I have studied Eastern mysticism and philosophies, so I was open to the idea that the spine is of key importance. Paul Bragg told me

"Look to the spine." He told me that if your spine is rigid, tight, and crooked, then your life is as well.

I have had a long interest in the spine and I've actually seen how important it is with clients and patients over the years. For example, a young boy who was in a coma for 3-1/2 years came out of it after I adjusted him. People who were paralyzed and quadriplegics responded tremendously under my care. I saw so many amazing things that it was undeniable that the spine was one of the most important structures of the body.

The body is designed with such wisdom that it protects the most important elements. Obviously, the brain is number one, the heart is second, the lungs are third, and the spinal column — an extension of the brain — is right there with them. Those are the most vital organs of survival and the body keeps them in complete mobility and houses them within a structure of protection.

The brain and spine together are like the golden rod of our existence and chiropractic allows for full expression of life by removing interferences to the functioning of those most delicate structures.

How does chiropractic offer people an opportunity to realize an enhanced quality of life?

I am a firm believer that if everybody who went to a chiropractor measured their income levels before and after a year's worth of care, most would see an increase in their incomes. For some, it might remain the same but for most the overall increase in productivity and income would more than pay the cost of their care. It would actually be an investment.

I know some people who were in really precarious situations with their spines and health but once they started getting adjustments their productivity at work went up, they started to have more confidence, and they made more money. They valued themselves, saved money, started entrepreneurial adventures, and ended up building businesses that made four to six times the income they had originally! I am certain that chiropractic protocols and procedures assisted them in their businesses and economics.

What do you feel has happened to the chiropractic profession that may have limited it from being seen by the world in its true nature?

Chiropractors — not all of them, but many — have really dug deep and explored their own philosophy to such a degree they are inspired by the depths of it. Yet, some have subordinated themselves to other health professions, minimized themselves as chiropractors, and exaggerated the importance of other health care fields and models.

When you do that, you tend to inject the values and beliefs of those other professions into chiropractic instead of allowing the genius, uniqueness, and magnificence of our chiropractic concepts to shine. True chiropractic visionaries are essential periodically to clean out the brush and light the fire to make the forest grow again. That has been a challenge at times, because people don't always probe deeply enough into the magnificence of our profession's principles to realize what we are contributing. Some of the greatest scientists, biologists, physiologists, and Nobel Prize winners have acknowledged the presence of Innate Intelligence and the body's wisdom and healing power. We don't fully appreciate the plasticity of the brain and the adaptability of the mind and sometimes, as a result, we subordinate ourselves to other schools of thought. The key is to be strong and allow the original genius and authenticity of our profession to keep shining.

Chiropractic has become tagged as a pain relief specialty. In your opinion what more does it have to offer people?

The truth is not in the hands of the masses but always in the hearts of the masters. The masters must pursue the wisdom regardless of what people are expecting. If we let children run the profession or let children run the professors at universities, we'd all probably just be watching TV. The professor has to guide the direction of the masses and educate the kids, you might say. Chiropractic is definitely more that just a pain reliever

Chiropractic has a major contribution to make to the world: ensuring that people's spines and physiology are congruent and functioning at maximum potential. We have a major contribution to make to society — if we just stick to our principles.

What is the purpose of the chiropractic adjustment and how does not receiving chiropractic care impact one's life?

There is no way human beings can maximize their potential if their spines and articulations — are subluxated. If the spine is not fully mobile and doesn't have a full range of motion, impulses from the brain will be impeded and physiology will be affected. We cannot maximize our potential as long as subluxations dominate. Having the spine periodically evaluated, mobilized, and adjusted maximizes human life.

It's like my oldest chiropractic saying, "Minimize subluxation and maximize the expression of life." I've been in practice and studying chiropractic now for 31 years. I've seen people in their 50s who were injured in their 20s and 30s, and their spinal degeneration is already starting because no one took care of them at the time of injury. There's no doubt that adjusting the spine and keeping it aligned increases the probability of having less degeneration and more potential in all areas of life.

What is your favorite quote and how has it impacted your life?

I have a number of quotes. I could give you thousands of them. One of them is: "The universe is my playground, the world is my home, every country is a room in the house, and every city is another platform to share my heart, soul, message, and inspiration with people around the world."

Others are, "I'm always at the right place at the right time to meet the right people to experience the right moment of love." And "I am a master healer, whoever I touch becomes healthy and inspired." One Paul Bragg gave me when I was 17 goes, "I am a genius and I apply my wisdom."

How is chiropractic unique and what does it offer that other health professions do not?

Many models in the healing arts rely on the idea that you don't have any power and need outside things to give you power. The thing that I love about chiropractic — and that brought tears to my eyes when I read "The Chiropractic Story" — was that there is truly a power that made the body that heals the body. Anyone who studies the laws of the universe and physiology to the depth that they are humbled by it will come to realize the wisdom in the body. It's just amazing.

I was at the Institute of Advanced Studies in Princeton and I had the opportunity to spend time with Freeman J. Dyson, who took over Albert Einstein's position in 1955 as professor emeritus. I had a nice chat with him for a few hours and we talked about biology, Innate Intelligence, and other things. This is one of the top minds in the world and he totally understood, acknowledged, and believed that there was a field of intelligence that governed biology. The brightest minds on the planet have this awareness.

I think chiropractic contributes to that awareness in the world. Pioneers live on the edge of the known and the unknown. The unknown is always sort of a mystical journey and the known is always an historical journey. We have to make sure that the mysteries and the histories are constantly growing.

I think chiropractic is at the forefront of bringing about acknowledgement of that mystery and of the intelligence that governs it. We use our own Innate Intelligence — through chiropractic adjustments — to direct the power through the body and allow it to work.

Remember the boy who was in a coma? He hadn't moved or been conscious for more than three years and I adjusted his spine and released that power from his brain. I watched him come around, move his body, start to make noise, and speak. I observed amazing things happen. I witnessed a spine go from not allowing full expression to, all of a sudden, doing just that. It's awe inspiring.

What do you sense was the intention behind the creation of chiropractic?

I think D.D. Palmer, a pioneer who had studied various forms of healing and personal development including magnetism, was a thoughtful individual and wanted to know the answers to things. When he had the experience with Harvey Lillard, he wanted to then find out why and how that thrust on his spine made a difference and allowed Lillard to regain his hearing.

Early on, he was an anatomy and physiology buff and he wanted to find out more about how and why hearing could be restored, in case there was something new he could bring to the world. Pioneers love answering questions, solving problems, investigating mysteries, and tackling challenges. Palmer was one of those individuals. We are here today because of a man like that, someone who was willing to explore the unknown to contribute something novel and great for humanity.

Who are some of your mentors and what impact have they had on your life?

There are piles of them. When I was in chiropractic college, I met an Indian gentleman named Lakishwar Ram who introduced me to the deeper mysteries of life and the exploration of many different fields. He had multiple PhDs. and was a very bright man. I can say thank you to him because he inspired my life.

Obviously, when I graduated, Jim Parker had an influence on my life. I started speaking at Parker when I was in my late 20s.

I've been blessed to read nearly 29,000 books over the last 37 years. I have just devoured literature from every imaginable walk and field of life. I read every day so there are thousands of authors who have influenced me. The great Greek philosophers, the Western mystics, the great theologians, and the great writers in almost every field, from business to politics, have impacted me. I have been interested in studying the lives and teachings of just about anyone who has left an immortal legacy in the world. They are all my mentors.

What are some things, if any, you have had to give up in order to devote your life to chiropractic?

I don't think of "giving up" anything; I think of transforming everything. I don't think in terms of gain and loss. I frequently say that a master lives in a world of transformation and never with the illusion of gain and loss.

I love what I do and nothing feels like sacrifice. I love watching people when the light bulb goes on and their eyes open and they see the mission they want to dedicate their lives to: doing something extraordinary, magnificent, and inspiring.

I love watching people heal. I was giving chiropractic care yesterday in Calgary. A lady was having problems with her intestines and the right side of her body. I was blessed to have the knowledge of chiropractic adjusting and reflex testing. I was very grateful that I had those tools and that inspires me. Any time you can make a difference in someone else's life, you have fulfillment.

I love watching people when the light bulb goes on and their eyes open and they see the mission they want to dedicate their lives to: doing something extraordinary, magnificent, and inspiring.

I study every day so I can offer ideas and services that make a difference. Most people want their lives to be easy but as they search for ways to make it easier, they actually make their lives more difficult. The wise person finds challenges, problems, and difficulties in the world and looks for solutions. As they seek out problems and difficulties, they find solutions that make their life easy.

What turns you on creatively, spiritually, or emotionally?

Doing what I love doing every day — researching, writing, traveling, teaching, and bringing healing. I dedicate every single day of my life to doing that. I was asked last night, "What do you do for chilling out and vacation?" I said, "Well my life is a vacation and I really don't think about it." I don't get up in the morning thinking about how I want to go on a vacation. I love what I do too much to take a break from it!

Where do you see the profession 10 years from now?

When people ask me that, I usually say that leaders will tell me where they're taking it and followers will ask me where it's going. The real truth is it will go wherever the leaders of our profession take it. It can go in a different direction tomorrow with a different leader. If you don't like where today's leaders are taking it, become a more powerful leader so you can take it where you would love it to go.

I made a commitment when I graduated from chiropractic college. I stood up to speak on graduation day and I said I am going to make sure that the deep philosophy of chiropractic stays alive as long as I am alive and I am going to keep sharing that message. Whether I am talking to businesses, leaders, football teams, soccer teams, celebrities, and wherever I go around the world visiting various countries, I still share the principles of chiropractic.

What do you mean by the deep philosophy of chiropractic?

The universe is basically a mixture of energy and matter and without question the expression of that is what we call life. Energy without matter is expressionless and matter without energy is motionless — the two together make up the existence of conscious life.

We in the chiropractic profession are working with that energy in the sense that when we align the spine, we actually allow that energy to fully maximize its expression in the form of physiology and homeostasis. We have a number of feedback mechanisms in the body and when we adjust the spine, we allow the feedback systems to do their job.

One of the grandest realizations we have is that there is an intelligence in the universe. I present a seminar program called The Breakthrough Experience pretty much every weekend of my life where people get to experience what Innate Intelligence is. I help them experience this homeostatic function in their own psychology, physiology, and sociology. They see it and when they do they're awestruck because they realize that we really do live in a field of intelligence governing life. Chiropractic is basically a science, art, and philosophy expressing that profound truth on earth.

What profession other than your own would you like to have attempted?

I'm a Renaissance man, so I have been blessed to speak on atomic physics, astronomy, theology, and philosophy. I was recently asked to speak at Salem University to 3,000 kids on philosophy. I have spoken at Harvard and I have been blessed to travel around the world to speak on many different topics. I like to be able to study the laws of the universe in every field and discipline and share whatever inspires. I consider myself a teacher, healer, and philosopher because of that.

Are there any other comments you'd like to share about the wonders of chiropractic?

The wisest thing we can do is give ourselves permission to be leaders and honor our professional principles and not subordinate ourselves to outside influences or think we are lacking something. The world treats us the way we treat ourselves. If we value ourselves, the world values us.

Some chiropractors don't value themselves as fully as they could if they explored, discussed, and discerned the wisdom of the chiropractic principles. I frequently say: "Don't shrink, shine. Don't be shallow, be deep!" Allow your message to go out to the world. Those with a mission have a message. Bring that message to the world. Speak up and share it.

Years from now when people look at your tombstone, what would you want them to read?

On the last day of your life, you're going to ask a simple question, "Did I do everything I could with everything I was given?" I want to be able to say, "Here lies a man who exemplified the human potential to its fullest. He did what he loved and loved what he did."

ॐ

John F. Demartini, D.C., is a chiropractor, human behavioral specialist, educator, and international authority on maximizing human awareness and potential. His studies encompass more than 270 different academic disciplines including research into most of the classical writings of both Orient and Occident.

He shares the synthesized messages of great world teachers from most major disciplines both past and present and provides answers and solutions to many of life's questions and challenges in more than 40 published books, 50 CDs/DVDs and 160 manuscripts.

As an educator, Dr. Demartini constantly travels the globe teaching students from all backgrounds and disciplines the workings of the universe, how to understand and transform social dynamics, and how to activate potential by understanding human nature.

To date, he has taught his principles and methodologies in 58 countries and has students in most countries across the world. Dr. Demartini is founder of the Demartini Institute, originator of the Demartini Method and he has homes in the United States, Australia, and on The World of ResidenSea.

Our task must be to free ourselves from this prison by widening our circle of compassion to embrace all living creatures and the whole of nature in its beauty.

Albert Einstein

Donny Epstein

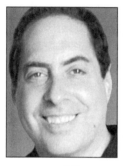

Where are you from originally and what was your childhood like?

I was born in Brooklyn, New York and I was an interesting child. I didn't speak until I was about 4 years old. They said I was developmentally delayed, at least that's the term they would use these days. Even as a child, I had a unique way of experiencing the world in that I saw energy, colors, forms, and sounds. I guess that was natural for teenagers in the '60s, but I had that experience as a kid — and without the drugs!

Somehow, I saw this energetic connection between things and people and I have to admit it was very scary because there was no context for that. I just basically stifled those experiences because of that lack of context. I was a very creative kid, yet slow in most things and, being labeled developmentally delayed, I did not believe I was smart.

I did have points of amazing transcendent awareness — that's the best way I can describe it — that didn't fit in with being a "slow" kid. By the time I was 17, I started having a more normal, or a more *culturally* normal way of experiencing the world.

What inspired you to get involved with chiropractic?

I was in my third year at Brooklyn College and I was going to apply for a new master's program at NYU for physiotherapy. I thought I'd end up in research in physiotherapy because my model of the world at that time was really clear — that the nervous system pretty much stored things in an interesting way.

Holographic was not a term for it then, but the premise was that the whole body stored information about everything. I knew that alternative methods, perhaps in physiotherapy, would help people develop alternative strategies for healing. However, the day I was sending my money order to NYU, my dad stopped me and said, "You are not going to apply to get a master's in the physiotherapy program; you are going to become a chiropractor."

He'd just seen my cousin, Arthur Pine, a chiropractor whose son was on the faculty at Columbia Institute of Chiropractic, and was told that the school was expanding. Pine suggested that I apply right away because I'd be automatically accepted.

I checked out what chiropractic was and its philosophy really interested me. I enrolled in the school, read about chiropractic, visited chiropractors in the area, got under chiropractic care, and that's how it all started.

Where do you currently reside and how are you spending your time these days?

I don't know where I reside but home is wherever my heart is and wherever my wife is. I collect my mail in Boulder, Colorado. The way we travel and the way our relationships are, we had to redefine what we call home and family.

I've spent my time developing Network Spinal Analysis for the chiropractic arena, Somato Respiratory Integration for the lay public and chiropractic profession, and the model of The Twelve Stages of Healing. I teach all of those things and just developed Reorganizational Healing, which is a meta-model of all of my life work to date (featured in the May 2009 issue of *Journal of Alternative and Complementary Medicine*).

The model's premise is that rather than trying to restore an individual's previous state, we can reorganize it to a higher level of complexity. It's not about the symptomatic parts of his or her body changing; it's about reorganizing his or her life. We're very much involved in the research agenda with this and other areas. I have a new discipline that I'll be starting to teach soon, which is inspired by what we have found in my past 30 years of experience and through our understanding of a whole new realm of informational fields around the body. These new models and paradigms on informational fields help give meaning to a person's life on a whole, wide, new range.

I'm also involved with many meetings on different levels dealing with cultural initiatives with people who are offering new ideas on the human condition and situation, and building bridges between them.

Chiropractic philosophy is not just about chiropractic. Chiropractic adopted the philosophy from life and other types of philosophies as part of its package in reference to the vertebral subluxation.

Expanding on the philosophies and doing basic science research that demonstrates certain things that are congruent with the original chiropractic tenants, as well as further out has been a passion of mine.

How does the profession differ now from when you first became involved?

Right now, the chiropractic profession doesn't have any particular identity. It's a profession in search of one. It's a very dangerous place to be. Right now, chiropractic is in its winter. When I got involved, chiropractic was in its autumn. In autumn, you could do anything and people would just show up. We could talk about our philosophy and they would sign up for care. It was amazing. In its autumn, you could sit there and the crops would just fall all over you.

Chiropractic is definitely in its winter and people need to understand this, but also understand that they can prepare by advancing their skills, going back to all of the fundamentals, remembering their vision, and getting ready for springtime when things can be wonderful.

Because chiropractic has lost its identity, the structure that insulates itself from change is weakened. There isn't even coherent agreement on chiropractic as a low back model. It's at a very dangerous point now, where chiropractic will either become allopathic or reinvent itself in a different way. To reinvent itself, the science, art, and philosophy have to be advanced with outcome assessments.

I went to Columbia Institute of Chiropractic, which became known as New York Chiropractic College when I graduated. We had to sign a document that said we were not going to practice medicine and we were not going to diagnose and treat disease. It was a different time, and coming from a straight perspective, we were told that doctors who took blood pressure were considered mixers.

Back then, unlike today, every course was taught by chiropractors. One of my biggest mentors at the time was Dr. Tom Whitehorne in the philosophy and technique departments. Dr. Reggie Gold had just left

> *Chiropractic is definitely in its winter and people need to understand this, but also understand that they can prepare by advancing their skills, going back to all of the fundamentals, remembering their vision, and getting ready for springtime when things can be wonderful.*

the school a few years before. That same year I graduated as one of the first graduates of the newly renamed New York Chiropractic College, Sherman College of Straight Chiropractic graduated its first class and Reggie was there in the philosophy department.

There was an explosion at that time in chiropractic and it was experiencing a summer-to-autumn season. So many new techniques were created, Parker Seminars were huge and were filling up Madison Square Garden and the Felt Forum, and all these new methods were coming out in the profession.

When I went to school, we had four semesters of chiropractic philosophy with Stephenson's textbooks and essays. I had a year of instrumentation and a year of full-spine technique including Toggle Recoil. I had a year of Gonstead technique, a year of SOT technique, a year of Applied Kinesiology, and we started adjusting in the second semester but first we used instrumentation to see what the temperature break was.

Most chiropractic practices were cash practices and everyone got excited talking about the philosophy of chiropractic. That was good enough for patients to come in and sign up for care.

We were told to find the primary subluxation and the magic would be in our chiropractic analysis, which led me to eventually develop Network Spinal Analysis as a continuation of what I learned in school. I had learned about checking the different systems by helping the areas of the vertebral-dural relationships and taking care of those first before addressing anything else.

When I went to chiropractic college, insurance wasn't a big thing in chiropractic. In New York State, we didn't even have insurance reimbursement. Most chiropractic practices were cash practices and everyone got excited talking about the philosophy of chiropractic. That was good enough for patients to come in and sign up for care.

Now, things have changed. People don't want to be sold things; they don't want to buy a philosophy anymore. They want to know what works and about your definitive outcome assessments. They also want something that their social network supports. They want to research the methodology of what we're doing; they want practical stuff.

When I got out of school, no one would have ever thought to ask for a second opinion in medicine. In the 1980s, people began to ask for second opinions. Now, the person first checks online for information and he or she comes into the office knowing more about multiple influences on health than the practitioner!

Practitioners today need to be savvy and able to know if they're producing results. They have to know what outcomes they're looking for. If they're going to offer long-term care, they have to know that their patients haven't just leveled off and are being maintained there. Are they still improving and what does improving mean? Technology makes different tools — from Surface EMG and thermograph units to heart rate variability, posture analysis, and computerized X-ray units — available to the chiropractor to answer these questions.

Research shows that the individual is the only one who knows if he or she is truly "well." Wellness is about our self-perception of how we're doing through different domains. The practitioner knows there is no relationship at all between a person's symptoms and whether or not he or she is ill. You could be ill and have no symptoms and be well with symptoms. The really powerful question isn't, "How do you feel?" but "How do you believe you're doing?" or even better, "How do you feel about how you feel?"

How does chiropractic relate to a person realizing his or her fullest human potential?

I really have a challenge with the concept of "fullest human potential" because to me it's often reduced to a bunch of New Age crap. If chiropractors really believe they release full potential, it's essential they have outcomes assessments so they can see a person's baseline and then determine if they're improving. I think it's time for the "chiropractic chiropractor" to stop hiding behind the rhetoric if the clinical results are not happening.

I don't know what a person's full potential is. The practitioner needs to start looking at what full potential really means. My mission in life has been to find out what the structure would be for people who were Innately guided, who were more passionate, loving, and creative. What would the spine have to be for them to be that way? What would the nervous system be like? How would they talk and what would their linguistic patterns be? How would their spines be different from everyone else's and what patterns would they show?

There is a relationship between perception, behavior, and structure. For any given structure of the body, there's a certain behavior. If your neck and shoulders are forward, you have to have a relationship with anger. If you neck is rigid with loss of curves, you are going to have the tendency to be stoic and not feel as much. If you live your life being depressed or angry, in order to maintain that state your spine is going to have to position and lock itself into anger or depression.

On the other hand, people who are loving and totally accepting of life have more flexible curves in their spine, the chest rises up more, and breath patterns are different. Perception and behavior will mimic structure and structure will mimic behavior.

Chiropractors deal with the relationship of structure and we need to determine how influencing the structure influences people's perceptions, the way they experience the world, the emotions they have, their behaviors, and the actions they take. By intervening in the structure of the system, a chiropractor can influence the individual to express a greater level of his or her potential by also being able to shift perception and behavior.

Perception and behavior will mimic structure and structure will mimic behavior.

This led me to develop Network Spinal Analysis and we have conducted or now have research going on at six major universities (a seventh is coming online soon) to study the neurological wave of the spine under Network care and how it organizes at higher levels of complexity as care progresses. Papers are coming out on how this somatic wave moves through the spine in the course of care, how the structure of the spine shifts, how the behavior of the spine shifts, and how the vertebrae oscillate at different waves that can be seen and measured on the Surface EMG. We can actually demonstrate a reorganization or evolution of the human nervous system through a change in structure and behavior. This is how we see people reaching their potential.

We have also been able to demonstrate wave movements in the body that are consistent with what B.J. Palmer called the Human Carrier or Pulsation Wave. He said there is a nerve force carrier wave, which — if it can be expressed — can merge a person's Innate and educated into one.

He was looking through the oscillation and waves, trying to put all of them on one oscilloscope to find one wave pattern. We can now also demonstrate that a wave goes through the spine in the Network application of chiropractic care, called a Somatopsychic wave.

It appears to be unique for each individual, although there are definite common properties. Each person seems to have a mathematical algorithm for how the spine organizes itself. Adjusting the spine at certain vertebral-dural relationship areas with gentle touches cues the body to access authentic innate strategies to organize itself.

This is the key element. Chiropractic, according to D.D. Palmer and then B.J., was based on the principle that there is an organizing force in the universe and progression is a natural state.

I've spent my life looking into that. What would it look like if the spinal system reorganized? How could the body use these innate forces and how could it create the force of its own adjustment? How can we assess whether the system is organizing at higher levels? If, by adjusting vertebral subluxations, a person's Innate Intelligence is expressing itself more effectively, the system is indeed moving toward a greater level of potential. It isn't going to be in defense and fighting; it isn't going to be trying to protect itself anymore. It is going to be more creative and able to open the circle of perception to other people. It's going to be happier and going to come up with more creative solutions.

Right now I'm spending my time and energy looking at expanding the models we're speaking about, creating paradigms for all disciplines. The chiropractic niche is the chiropractic adjustment in relationship to these models. When you talk about increasing the innate potential within a person, I say that model worked in the '80s. At that time I said, "What would the spine look like if people were in fact living this type of life and how could I help that happen?" I realized that as long as I'm going to try and correct, fix, or maintain something, I'm still practicing the application of medicine.

Chiropractic has become tagged as a pain relief specialty. In your opinion what more does it have to offer people?

Number one, it comes back to this: is your objective restorative therapeutics or reorganizational healing? In restorative therapeutics, the concept is that the symptom or condition — or even the subluxation — messed up a person's life and made them uncomfortable and the adjustment is supposed to make that person comfortable.

The only thing is, I have no intention of taking away pain because without pain there's no motivation for change. Pain tells people to stop whatever they're doing immediately, take an inventory and self-assess, and make an instantaneous behavioral change. That is always what pain means in every case. It's an evolutionary mechanism.

The vertebral subluxation is the body's way of locking you into one perspective until you're able to finally be present with an experience. The subluxation stops you from fully feeling it and it disassociates you from it. As long as the pain is seen as an enemy or something you want to get rid of, you're going to have more of it in your life.

While pain promotes change, only a change in your identity — who you believe you are — will create progress. Your identity is locked in by your spine; your identity, your self defense, who you believe you are, your habitual emotions, your habitual patterns. All of these habituations are locked in by sensory motor elements of the spine. The emotional brain controls the excitability of every sensory motor neuron in the body. The purpose of emotion is to take immediate action and not think about it. Most people's pain comes from not taking the action they need. Through the structure, there is a signal and perception that people are not listening to. They're not making the necessary behavioral changes, and it hurts. If they were to experience a greater range of emotion, which is associated with a greater range of motion also, they would take different actions and the cycle would shift. One of the things that would be shifting is the subluxation pattern.

What is the purpose of the chiropractic adjustment?

The purpose of the chiropractic adjustment is to cue the brain and the body's self-organizing wisdom to observe itself and develop new energy efficient strategies for expressing its core nature. As that nature is maximized, the person evolves to the next level.

What do you sense was the intention behind the creation of chiropractic?

At the time D.D. Palmer created chiropractic, magnetism, "spirit", and energy fields were important matters. New inventions were coming out and people were talking theories of relativity; the relationship between energy and matter and function, the speed of light. I believe the original concept of chiropractic was the concept of tone, which is the same concept we are coming back to now — that everything oscillates.

D.D. said that everything was founded upon tone and that molecular oscillation is the basis of consciousness. I believe chiropractic was originally formed as a means of treating the spinal system, through the nervous system, to allow the individual to evolve on this plane and on other levels of consciousness.

D.D. also said that consciousness comes from absolute planes as well as other planes and that you are creating an oscillatory field with individuals and humanity. That was the original concept, but there was no social construct for it. If there is no cultural context for it, it gets put into whatever limited context you have. When B.J. Palmer further developed it, he made it into more of a health system because health was the closest thing they had, but I don't think health was really at all what it was developed for.

The profession would have been a lot different if it had been developed based on what we now know. It would have been developed as a means of advancing the physical embodiment of consciousness for individuals, community, and society. I want to be clear that I do not believe the original intention of chiropractic was to be what it is now. Can chiropractic be practiced as it was originally intended? I don't believe that the current doctor of chiropractic can practice in that original way and be in compliance with state law in most jurisdictions.

What do you feel has happened to the chiropractic profession that may have limited it from being seen by the world in its true nature?

Chiropractors have totally dropped the ball on chiropractic, period. It's real simple. Any discipline needs demonstrable outcomes. If you say that chiropractic is about improving one's potential, what outcome assessments do you use before and after individual visits to show this? What specifically are you looking for?

Chiropractic has become, and in reality is, a legal and political entity — it's what the schools teach and what the state boards test for. That has nothing to do with what the promise of chiropractic is. The only way we can fulfill that promise is for all chiropractors to be honest and ask themselves: "How do I know what I'm doing is working?" and "How do my patients know if it's working?"

By no means am I suggesting that chiropractors are wrong with what they do or that they are somehow missing the boat, but rather the profession as a whole has been asleep and we need to reorganize the structure of the profession in order to evolve it and the people we touch. When you're fighting for your life you don't grow.

Who are some of your mentors and what impact have they had on your life?

My mentor in chiropractic college was Dr. Tom Whitehorne, who was my upper cervical practitioner, my philosophy instructor, and my technique instructor at the Columbia Institute of Chiropractic. He held firm to the philosophy and he helped me understand that either chiropractic is specific or it's something else.

Another was Dr. Pasquale Cerasoli, who made a statement to me when I was in my more dogmatic fundamentalist chiropractic phase and was telling everyone I adjusted by hand only. He said to me, in that wonderfully sincere way, "Donald, do you just adjust by your hand or do you use your heart?" He told me to read D.D. Palmer and understand the concept of tone and until I did that I was missing the boat. So, he would be another hero.

Another was Dr. Jim Parker, who introduced most of the major innovative techniques in chiropractic at Parker Seminars — the low-force techniques, emotional-centered techniques, SOT, Applied Kinesiology, NET, BEST, NSA, and more. One of the many things that Jim Parker represented was that first you were a spiritual healer and you must accept that all healing is spiritual or it is not healing.

Another early hero of mine was Dr. Vern Pierce. He, along with Dr. Glenn Stillwagon, helped me understand the importance of assessing spinal outcomes on a dynamic level.

A couple of others are Dr. Jim Sigafoose, who's a hero and always an inspiration for his ability to compassionately and joyously celebrate the principle of chiropractic, and Dr. Arno Burnier, a peer of mine who practiced Network Spinal Analysis years ago and actually taught many of the seminars during those first years.

Dr. Reggie Gold is also a hero, for his ability to tell the chiropractic story and be a guiding force as one of chiropractic's warriors. Another I must mention is Dr. Gerry Clum, because he's the person who suggested I take a look at health-related quality of life assessments. He told me I'm looking not so much at chiropractic assessments as social science assessments and that I need to look at what social scientists said.

Another is Dr. Christopher Kent, who's been an amazing friend and influence. He, along with Dr. Patrick Gentempo, has the ability to integrate science, art, and philosophy and to see how the little things we do affect the bigger picture in different ways.

I must also mention my wife, Dr. Jackie Knowles Epstein. When I met her, I was going to stop teaching chiropractic and just continue in private practice but she helped me to bridge the gap between my head and my heart and realize that it isn't about chiropractic or about me and my technique, but it's about the call of humanity and future generations. She's still the single strongest force and light of my life.

Are there any other comments you'd like to share about the wonders of chiropractic?

We have a short time for the chiropractic profession to either die and be replaced by another form of manipulative therapy or to evolve into what is needed for the future of humanity. That's going to require practitioners to ask themselves how they can step up and do more for people *this month* than they have for the entire past year. How can they see the person and not the subluxation? How can they focus not on the imprisonment of the spine but the liberation of humanity? And how do they know if it's working?

There will be pressure put on the profession to supply the public with what it wants rather than what the profession wants to supply the public with. If we make it past the next couple of years, I believe there is really a chance.

Years from now when people look at your tombstone, what would you want them to read?

Donny Epstein: here lies a Mensch. For those who don't know what a Mensch is, it's a Yiddish term, which means a good person who does the right thing for the right reason without being asked, no matter the cost.

For the past three decades, **Donny Epstein, D.C.,** has been at the forefront of the global wellness movement. He is the founder and developer of Somato Respiratory Integration and Network Spinal Analysis, as well as the developer of Reorganizational Healing, and an Emerging Energetic based discipline.

His books include "The Twelve Stages of Healing," "Healing Myths, Healing Magic" and "The Boomerang Principle." His methods have been featured on television as well as in numerous magazines and newspapers around the world. His work has also been published extensively in professional journals.

Dr. Epstein, a 1977 graduate of New York Chiropractic College, established two successful wellness practices in New York before relocating to Colorado and committing to full time research, development, and instruction.

In the early '80s, he began teaching wellness programs, which he now teaches internationally to thousands of individuals annually. Dr. Epstein serves on the science board of the Angelicum Center in Milan, a think-tank dedicated to helping advance human dignity, compassion and respect.

The vast majority of human beings dislike and even actually dread all notions with which they are not familiar... Hence it comes about that at their first appearance innovators have generally been persecuted and always derided as fools and madmen.

Aldous Huxley

Thom Gelardi

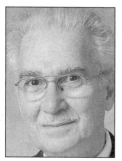

Where are you from originally and what was your childhood like?

I was born and raised in Mount Vernon, New York. While I didn't realize it then, looking back we would have been considered poor. My father was a sign painter and my mother worked in a sweatshop. Life was good for my three sisters and me. Mother and dad kept worrisome things away from us, but they had much to worry about, particularly finances and my health, which among other things was a great financial burden on the family. Through the example of my parents and the culture at that time, we learned much about love, honesty, the work ethic, and being happy.

What inspired you to get involved with chiropractic?

I was inspired to become a chiropractor first through my experience under medicine and then as a chiropractic patient. I was a very sickly child, spending my first eight birthdays in the hospital and continuing to be in the hospital every year or two until discovering chiropractic at 17. One of those early stays in the hospital involved my spending two and a half years in bed. I took medicine every day of my life until my first visit to a chiropractor.

I was diagnosed with a number of different conditions, but the main one was rheumatic fever. It soon became bacterial endocarditis (bacteria caused inflammation of the lining of the heart), which in turn caused a heart murmur. Most frustrating was the lack of an answer to the question, "Why me?" It seemed as though microorganisms just randomly selected victims. I lived in the same house with other members of the family, ate the same foods, breathed the same air, etc. In fact, I was looked after more carefully than were the others. If there was something different about me, why weren't they treating *me* instead of the bacteria?

When I was 17, my brother-in-law — who suffered with migraine headaches and found help through chiropractic — urged me to see a chiropractor for my heart condition. I told him that my murmur was caused from scar tissue on heart valves, and just as nothing would remove scar tissue from the skin, nothing would remove it from a heart valve. He continued to insist that I see a chiropractor, so I went to please him.

I quickly told the chiropractor why he couldn't help me. He somewhat agreed that perhaps my body could not rebuild a damaged valve, but he asked me if I thought improved general health might make a weak heart function somewhat better or last longer. I had to agree. What he said next was my epiphany. He said our bodies have an innate striving to create and maintain their own health. I can't tell you how strongly that resonated with what was probably my subconscious belief system.

He said that the body's adaptive mechanisms were carried out by the nervous system. It transmitted organizing and coordinating information, in the form of mental impulses, from the brain to all parts of the body. He went on to say that bacteria are always in the body but rather than **causing** disease, they become pathogenic as a **result** of sick and dying tissue. The "body's innate striving" bit profoundly affected me. It set me on fire.

He explained how vertebral subluxation interferes with the body's innate striving to function normally and adapt to its environment. That was a plausible answer to my "why me" question — if there really was such a thing as a vertebral subluxation. I particularly liked the idea that the problem was about the functioning of my body and not an environment to which everyone else was adapting.

Even as a very young boy, I had always wondered why my body couldn't run itself. I didn't know if the chiropractor was right or wrong about subluxation, and while he didn't promise anything, he certainly pressed the right buttons. He also said that the body, when functioning at a high level, often could adapt or compensate for permanently damaged or missing parts. It was another reasonable idea and pressed another right button. I believed fully in what he said about how the body functioned and adapted to its environment, about the nervous system carrying information that controlled and coordinated function and that health was a state where the parts of the body functioned normally. I also believed he was a person of intelligence and integrity. I can't say I was convinced about vertebral subluxations or vertebral adjustments. That came later.

The chiropractor examined my spine and found that the top vertebra was subluxated. I had mixed feelings when I left his office, but most of them were good. On the positive side, he never listened to my heart or examined any part of me other than my spine. I was tired of the old and failed medical ceremony, with its stethoscopes, cardiograms, and prescription pads. This new ceremony gave me new hope.

On a less positive side, I thought there were plenty of honest medical doctors and much medical research being done and if there were anything to the subluxation theory, they certainly would have discovered it. The positives slightly outweighed that negative, and I felt I had nothing to lose but some money. So, on my own, I immediately quit taking all of my medications. I never liked taking medicine.

My health didn't noticeably change the first year but I wasn't sick or absent from school and I was no worse off for having stopped taking medicine. I tell chiropractic students that I continued chiropractic for three reasons. First, the chiropractor radiated good things: a rational philosophy, humanity, and integrity. Second, his explanations resonated with me and made more sense than anything I had ever heard. I would always go to the office loaded with questions and his answers always

The patients in his reception room, unlike those in medical offices, were all upbeat and sharing their stories about getting well from all sorts of health problems after traditional methods had failed.

seemed to be rational. Third, he was affordable. Maybe there was a fourth reason: The patients in his reception room, unlike those in medical offices, were all upbeat and sharing their stories about getting well from all sorts of health problems after traditional methods had failed. Some had back problems but the majority of the patients had chronic physiological problems: asthma, diabetes, skin conditions, epilepsy, etc.

I am now 75 years old and have not had so much as an aspirin since that first visit to the chiropractor. I have never missed a day of school or work since that first visit. My wife and I raised five children, all of whom were born at home. Other than one daughter who had a cut chin stitched up and a son getting a broken ankle set, we have all enjoyed great health with no medical or drug interventions.

I was inspired to become a chiropractor by chiropractic's vitalistic view of life, by the benefits I received and saw others receive. I continue to be excited about chiropractic because I've seen so many people enjoy better health. It's so refreshingly different than the Newtonian, mechanistic view of today's society. We are starting to hear more about "going green" and the value of organic foods, but chiropractic is more comprehensive. Chiropractic is more than adjusting an offending vertebra; it is a rational approach to living an ethical lifestyle as an integral part of nature.

Where do you currently reside and how are you spending your time these days?

After I graduated from chiropractic college, I followed one of my professors, Dr. Lyle W. Sherman, who was going into semi-retirement, to South Carolina. I live in Gaffney, South Carolina and after 50 years of practice, founding Sherman College of Straight Chiropractic and serving as its president, I am now in semi-retirement. I continue a small chiropractic practice, write, lecture, enjoy time with my wife Betty, the children and grandchildren, watching sunrises and sunsets, listening to the birds sing, and watching the squirrels steal our pecans.

How does the profession differ now from when you first became involved?

When I first learned of chiropractic, the profession was 56 years old. Much about the profession has changed since then, and most of the differences resulted from two major changes, one good and one not so good. On the good side, there is somewhat less harassment of the profession today from organized medicine and, because of that, less discrimination from governmental agencies. This has allowed the profession to serve more people and offer a sought-after career opportunity.

When I was introduced to chiropractic, practicing chiropractic was still illegal in New York and several other states. On the way to gaining state licensure throughout the country, thousands of chiropractors went to jail for the civil disobedience of providing chiropractic care to members of the public. Many chiropractors, on being released from jail, would go back into practice, frequently to be jailed again. Many of the people who were helped through chiropractic formed organizations that fought for the licensure of chiropractors.

In 1976, the chiropractic profession brought legal action against the AMA for trying to drive it out of business. The case cost more than a million dollars and took more than 14 years to move through the lower courts and reach the US Supreme Court. The court found the AMA and its allied organizations guilty of conspiratorial action directed toward driving the chiropractic profession out of the health care marketplace.

Today, chiropractic can be practiced in all 50 states. It's recognized throughout the U.S. in public and private health care programs and in the armed services. Chiropractic education and research now are supported both federally and privately and chiropractic colleges and practitioners serve in most areas of the world.

On the downside, the profession seems to have lost sight of its purpose. The purpose of the profession — as stated by its founder and as it served as the standard by which the value of all the profession's activities was determined — is to contribute to patient health thorough the correction of vertebral subluxation. D.D. Palmer, the founder of the profession, wrote: "Chiropractic is a name I originated to designate the science and art of adjusting vertebrae. It does not relate to the study of etiology or any branch of medicine. Chiropractic includes the science and art of adjusting vertebrae — the know-how and the doing."

The profession would advance faster if it stopped insisting on being classified as an unlimited primary health care profession in the model of allopathic or osteopathic medicine, and saw itself more in the model of... a limited primary health care profession.

The profession was not intended to be the treatment of disease or any symptoms or pain. It was not meant to duplicate the services offered in the fields of medicine, meditation, nutrition, exercise or the myriad of other health disciplines. It was not intended as a cure for all things or some things. The profession would advance faster if it stopped insisting on being classified as an unlimited primary health care profession in the model of allopathic or osteopathic medicine, and saw itself more in the model of dentistry and optometry, a limited primary health care profession.

Palmer wrote: "Those who expect to put in a lifetime combating disease, fighting the entrance of disease, as tho it was an enemy with hostile intent, should not learn Chiropractic."

Subluxations were understood to be one of the major categories of interferences to the body's innate striving to maintain its own health. There are no symptoms directly associated with vertebral subluxation. Subluxations produce functional disharmony that gradually lowers resistance and increases susceptibility. They cause the body to be less able to adapt to its environment. The consequent disease depends on the location and kind of subluxation, one's genetic predisposition and the environment.

To gain legislative authority to adopt practices from other health care areas, the profession has had to include them as part of the chiropractic curriculum. In order to do that, studies and clinical practices related to chiropractic have had to be reduced. I believe a profession that is focused and deep better serves the public than one that is broad and shallow.

How do chiropractic and performance relate?

There are many kinds of performance. As one example, when you consider that 90 percent of the accidents happen to only 10 percent of the people, you realize that some people have difficulty performing motor skills without having an accident. I believe that such mal-performance is a sign of poor health. Is it due to an inability to focus, mental confusion, mental distraction, or kinesthetic malfunction (the brain not being aware of the body's position relative to its environment)?

> **Parents often tell me their children play together noticeably better or make significantly better grades in school after their subluxations have been corrected for a short period.**

Chiropractors correct the vertebral subluxation, knowing that the body is always better without this interference to the nervous system and knowing that healthier people always have higher resistance. They're more alert and perform better as parents, spouses, or friends. They perform better on the golf course or football field, in the gym and on the job. We all know that some days we perform better than other days. The more physically and mentally fit we are, the more often we have high-performance days. Tiger Woods has his chiropractor travel with him to tournaments, not to treat sickness or pain (he has a sports trainer for that). The chiropractor is there to see that he doesn't perform while subluxated. Major sports teams have chiropractors who help players obtain optimum performance.

Parents often tell me their children play together noticeably better or make significantly better grades in school after their subluxations have been corrected for a short period.

A person is comprised of millions of cells and many organs. Like the parts of an orchestra, the output of each part of the body must be coordinated and in harmony with the output of all of the other parts if there is to be harmony rather than noise, health rather than malfunction. The output of an orchestra is coordinated by a conductor while the output of the infinitely more complex body is coordinated by mental impulses that move from the brain to the tissue cells via the central nervous system.

The performance of a runner, actor, executive, administrator, teacher, salesperson, or rabbi reflects the performer's mind and body, the performer's state of health. A runner, when performing, must breathe in extra air. Breathing in extra air won't help if her heart isn't pumping that air to the rest of her body or if the blood vessels of the abdominal organs don't constrict and those of the skeletal muscles relax, or if her skin doesn't play its role in the regulation of body temperature, and if any of a thousand other adaptive changes don't take place.

It doesn't matter how strong and talented the members of a football team are. If they aren't functioning harmoniously with each other they won't meet the challenges on the field of play. The same principle applies to the functioning of the parts of the body. Think of the physical and mental dexterity and agility needed to perform with a musical instrument or a tennis racket. Those same principles of coordination and harmony apply to meeting any of life's physical or mental challenges. Consider but a very few challenges to which we are constantly adapting: gravity, pollens, microorganisms, social stresses, temperature, humidity, barometric pressure, light, sounds and smells, and radio waves. It's said that our bodies must adapt to more than 30,000 ever-changing environmental forces every second.

An overwhelming thought is that this interdependency isn't only about the parts of our body, but the parts of our universe. Oneness and wholeness is of the universe and all division is an artificial construct of man. Each living thing is a cell of the universe, interdependent with the activities of all other living things. The universe and the planet are alive. Our pulmonary and digestive systems extend far beyond our bodies, and so do our nervous system and other systems.

As people grow healthier, so do their thoughts, emotions, and activities. As we were designed to be physically healthy, so were we designed to be mentally and emotionally healthy. I tell my practice members that the chiropractor removes one major form of interference to their being well and they should examine their lives and remove other forms of interference. If all interferences are removed and healthy things (food, thoughts, air, activities, etc.) are put into the body, we will have a 99.44 percent chance of avoiding health problems. Health comes from within or not at all. As Michelangelo explained, David was already in the marble and to see David all he had to do was to remove that part of the marble that was blocking its appearance.

How does chiropractic relate to a person realizing his or her fullest human potential?

Ivan Illich defined health as that which allows a person to live most autonomously. None of us is completely autonomous, but the least dependent on supplements, antidepressants, antibiotics, pain pills, and other crutches that we can be, the greater the indication is that we are healthy.

While the United States has a higher percentage of its people on prescription crutches and spends more per capita on health care than any other nation in the world, it's one of the unhealthiest nations on earth. The greater our ability is to live autonomously, the greater our human potential. A healthy person is more curious and wanting to learn, more adventurous and wanting to explore, more of a reasonable risk-taker and wanting to advance. Healthy people are more alive, more aware of opportunities, and more willing and able to seize opportunities for success and security.

I must say, lest I be misunderstood, there's more to health than just being free of vertebral subluxation. There are other health concerns that are addressed by other people or should be addressed by each individual. I was about to say "addressed by other health care professions," but most other "health" care professions are more concerned with getting a disease or pain out of the body than getting health into it. Chiropractors don't fix teeth, fit glasses or set broken bones, but these are important concerns that when necessary should be addressed. A few of the other important concerns are knowledge of the principles relating to general exercise and nutrition. Everyone should study the laws of nature relating to the care of their bodies.

How does chiropractic offer people an opportunity to realize an enhanced quality of life?

Chiropractic offers people an enhanced quality of life in two major ways. Chiropractic is grounded in an evolving philosophy and chiropractors teach these philosophical or health principles to their patients. Principles are important because from one principle you can deduce an infinite number of practices in all areas of life. A profession's philosophy is its understanding of the fundamental nature of reality and man and man's relationship to the things of reality.

The philosophy of chiropractic is particularly concerned with the laws and principles of health. That applies to all kinds of health: physical, mental, economic, social, spiritual, etc. An example of a very simple but often overlooked principle is "use it or lose it." You might easily see its relationship to the skeletal muscles of the body but it also relates to the mind, the immune system, the ability to handle responsibility, the building of character, and much more.

The second way chiropractic offers people an opportunity to realize an enhanced quality of life is through the correction of a vertebral subluxation. Vertebral subluxation reduces one's creative potential, expression of virtue, and appreciation of beauty, all of which enhance life.

What do you feel has happened to the chiropractic profession that may have limited it from being seen by the world in its true nature?

The profession seems to have lost sight of its true purpose. It has failed to stay focused on its mission. It became distracted by political medicine's distorted charges that chiropractors were not as well educated and had a lower standard of practice than those of physicians. Chiropractic had a very high standard of education and practice relative to its mission. It did not have the same standard of education and practice as medicine, any more than engineers have the same education or standard of practice as musicians. But, rather than arguing the irrationality of political medicine's claim, political chiropractic abandoned the profession's mission and began making chiropractic education and practice more like that of medicine. It gave the profession a weird kind of bragging right at the cost of its mission. It had the pathos of the quote: "When you are up to your hind end in alligators, it is difficult to remember that your initial mission was to drain the swamp."

Granted, the road for chiropractic has been arduous. Deeply entrenched politically, overwhelmingly strong financially and having monopoly power socially, medicine and its allied professions and organizations — drug manufacturers, insurance companies, hospital associ-

> **Vertebral subluxation reduces one's creative potential, expression of virtue, and appreciation of beauty, all of which enhance life.**

ations, nurse associations ... and the heart, lung, cancer, spina-bifida, cerebral palsy associations, etc., etc. — were formidable foes for a young upstart profession.

Health insurance companies, because of the law, could not discriminate among health care providers. They could, however, cover or not cover certain procedures. To eliminate chiropractic, almost all insurance companies refused to recognize the vertebral subluxation as an abnormal condition. They would pay for spinal manipulation for the treatment of various conditions. To meet this challenge, political chiropractic and chiropractic trade associations again compromised the profession by obtaining legislation allowing chiropractors to practice treating disease and symptoms with spinal manipulation. This was rationalized as helping people afford chiropractic care, but it distorted not only the public's perception of chiropractic, but also that of the practitioner.

To eliminate chiropractic, almost all insurance companies refused to recognize the vertebral subluxation as an abnormal condition.

Chiropractic has become tagged as a pain relief specialty. In your opinion what more does it have to offer people?

Today's presentation of chiropractic is confusing. First, regardless of the value of pain relief, the objective of chiropractic is no more the relief of pain than it is the fitting of eyeglasses. Also, pain is a sign that the body is making an extra effort to maintain itself. Pain can result from the body trying to adapt to a very cold or hot environment, to high toxicity from something ingested or breathed, or from extra bright light causing the pupils of the eyes to quickly contract. Back pain may come when the back is healing from injury or is adapting to a certain posture. Pain directs our behavior. A pain in the shoulder or hip may tell us to move it carefully or not at all until the body repairs the damage. Pain also is very subjective and we can be conditioned to tolerate or abhor pain. Our attitude toward pain can lead to undesirable consequences. While pain from third degree burns over a considerable area of the body can cause life-threatening shock, there have been instances where, without the availability of an anesthetic, people have cut off their own hand, arm or leg in order to survive some accident, and they survived both the cutting and the pain. I am not advocating surgery without anesthesia, only pointing out that the body has a naturally high tolerance for pain. Our low pain tolerance comes from our culture, which in turn comes from drug company advertising that life should be without pain. In reality, we suffer more from this unnecessary masking of the body's healing methods and messages than we do from tolerating our everyday pains.

Again, relieving pain is not the purpose of chiropractic. Extreme pain should be medically evaluated and controlled.

What is the purpose of the chiropractic adjustment and how does not receiving chiropractic care impact one's life?

When a vertebra is subluxated, coordinating messages from the brain to the cells of the body are modified as they traverse nerve pathways in the area of the spine. These modified messages produce modified function or malfunction. The purpose of a chiropractic adjustment is to restore to normal the articulating relationship of a subluxated vertebra, removing the interference to the mental impulses.

Not receiving chiropractic care means having this nerve interference continue and having less than optimum health. It means less than complete mental, physical and social well-being. It means lowered resistance, lessened ability to heal, increased susceptibility and possibly pathology, and even death.

The World Health Organization defines health as more than the absence of disease — as complete mental, physical and social well-being. Health has to do with creativity, dexterity, awareness, self-confidence, the welcoming of healthy challenges, and much more. Disease is an artificial bureaucratic-made construct and not a reality in the sense of a cut, broken bone, burn, or subluxation. A disease is not an evil entity separate from the body that can be driven out with a poison or knife. A body that is malfunctioning is one that cannot adapt to everyday environmental forces, that can't adapt to the weather, pollens, bacteria, social stresses, etc.

Simply put, not receiving chiropractic care impacts one's life by keeping it from existing in full expression.

What is your favorite quote and how has it impacted your life?

I have many favorite quotes. In fact, Sherman College of Straight Chiropractic published a small book with about a hundred or so of my favorite quotes. It's called "Inspirations." With regard to health, I like a quote attributed to Socrates: "If there is one way better than another, it is the way of nature." I also like: "Health comes from within," and Shakespeare's: "The trouble dear Brutus is not in the stars, but in ourselves."

How is chiropractic unique and what does it offer that other health professions do not?

Chiropractic's uniqueness is its understanding of man's relationship to the things of existence, and its expounding on the practical applications of that knowledge for greater health, personal success, and the joy of living. It teaches that health comes from within and is not found outside the thing itself, i.e., in drugs, doctors, belief systems, charms, etc. It teaches that we have the choice of investing our time, intelligence and effort in health or in trying to manage our diseases and pain through pills, surgeries, and rituals.

Fighting disease is America's biggest and most profitable industry. Americans spend more than twice as much as any other country on legal drugs. The vast majority of Americans are taking legal drugs every day, and their health ranks near the bottom. The same legal drug attitude that has been engendered by our drug industry underlies our illegal drug problem. This same attitude of perfect health spills over to an attitude of perfect happiness. When we're not perfectly happy, too many look for a new situation or a pill.

Chiropractic is unique because of its unique mission. It's also one of the few voices that for more than a hundred years has been saying we cannot violate the laws of nature and expect to make things right by just taking a pill or confessing our sins. Nature is very just. We grow stronger by meeting the challenges of life. The things of nature stay in existence through tension and the tension of life is part of its joy.

What do you sense was the intention behind the creation of chiropractic?

Clearly, the founder of our profession stated that he created the chiropractic profession to bring the fruits of his discovery of the vertebral subluxation and its correction to the masses. He stated hundreds of times that chiropractic had one mission: to contribute to life and health through the correction of vertebral subluxation. He stated that chiropractic was not the practice of medicine or a therapy or treatment for any symptom, disease, or any condition other than vertebral subluxation.

Who are some of your mentors and what impact have they had on your life?

I have had, and now have, many mentors, most of them book authors. In chiropractic, the writings of the profession's founder, Daniel David Palmer and his son, Dr. B.J. Palmer have had a great influence on my life, not because of their authority but because of their rationality. Both Palmers had a clear and rational mission for the profession. B.J. Palmer greatly advanced the philosophy of chiropractic and — through his clinical research center — the science and art of chiropractic. Both Palmers loved the potential that existed in this new profession.

Dr. Lyle W. Sherman, the assistant director of B.J. Palmer's Research Center, was more than a colleague; he was my close friend. He greatly advanced my chiropractic knowledge and skills, for which I'll be forever grateful. I was impressed as much by his humility, his love for knowledge. He gave generously of himself to his patients, his profession, and his colleagues. He was a man who loved life, nature, people, and his work.

Mentors from my readings are many, including Ayn Rand, Rene Dubos, Mahatma Gandhi, Martin Luther King, Jr., Bahá'u'lláh, Aldous Huxley, Shakespeare, Saul Alinsky, and Ivan Illich.

What are some things, if any, you have had to give up in order to devote your life to chiropractic?

The only thing I gave up less than easily was not being able to spend more time with my wife, Betty, and our five children. Betty understood what I was trying to do and was as dedicated as I to advancing the profession and bringing its services to as many people as possible. The children also were supportive of our work but I missed much of their childhood. During my years as president of Sherman College of Straight Chiropractic, I also missed having a full practice. However, being one person, I chose my highest value and would do it the same today. I know what chiropractic could mean to this world and firmly believe what a Sherman trustee and mentor, Dr. Earl Powell, said about our need to advance the profession: "We are only rolling marbles, when we should be moving mountains."

What turns you on creatively, spiritually, or emotionally?

Being with honest, serving people who have a driving purpose and are pursuing it in an ethical manner.

Where do you see the profession 10 years from now?

I believe the profession stands on the brink of a precipice. To continue in its present, short-sighted direction of having an unnecessarily costly, burdensome, and in large measure superfluous therapeutic educational system designed more to impress than prepare practitioners to chiropractically serve, will cause its demise, as it did the demise of osteopathy. The profession's leaders should recognize the best way to glorify chiropractors is to fulfill our mission of bringing our unique service to the masses. Doing so would revolutionize not only health care but every aspect of society that depends upon the bodies and minds of its citizens.

What profession other than your own would you like to have attempted?

When I fly and I see the pilot, or go to see my accountant, lawyer, dentist or real estate sales person or developer, I sometimes ask myself how I would enjoy doing their work. The answer is always the same: I'd rather be a chiropractor. I found teaching at Sherman College very rewarding. I believe teaching particularly on the elementary and secondary level is probably life's highest calling, but that would be too big of a challenge for me. I am most thankful that I discovered chiropractic. It has allowed me great health, wonderful colleagues, and a work that I love.

New York native **Thom Gelardi, D.C.,** attended Palmer School of Chiropractic, where he studied under the legendary Dr. Lyle Sherman. After graduation in 1957, Dr. Gelardi opened an office in Gaffney, SC, to continue his mentorship with Dr. Sherman. In 1973, he founded Sherman College of Straight Chiropractic and served as its president until 1997, and then as chair of the board of trustees from 1997-2002.

Active in the South Carolina Chiropractic Association, he was that state's representative to the International Chiropractors Association, and started the South Carolina Chiropractic Research Bureau.

Dr. Gelardi's numerous honors and awards include: "Chiropractor of the Century" by the Federation of Straight Chiropractors and Organizations, a Fellow of the College of Straight Chiropractic, and "Chiropractor of the Year" by Sherman College in 1997.

Dr. Gelardi has traveled throughout the world as a lecturer and written extensively on chiropractic philosophy.

Patrick Gentempo

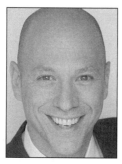

Where are you from originally and what was your childhood like?

I'm originally from New Jersey and I was brought up in Ramsey. I'm still in the same area right now. My upbringing was typical suburbia outside New York City. I come from an Italian family and both sides of grandparents are right from Italy. I had a pretty standard middle class upbringing. One of the highlights from childhood is that I was a five-time New Jersey State and two-time National AAU karate champion. I kind of walked to the beat of my own drum when I was a kid and had a mind of my own.

What inspired you to get involved with chiropractic?

I always felt I was going to be in health care. When I was growing up, I was very interested in reading how-and-why books about the human body and that kind of thing. Up until the mid-teens, I was pretty convinced I was going to medical school because heart surgery was something very interesting to me. I had experience in my mid-teens with a pretty significant health challenge. I was a wrestler in high school and during one match I bridged up on my neck, I felt my neck give, I had significant pain, muscle spasms, and what felt like swelling in there.

They picked me off the mat and brought me to a medical doctor who was a good guy. He did a very thorough evaluation and said that I had cervicalgia, myospasm, and inflammation. I asked him what those were and he said, "Neck pain, muscle spasm, and swelling." I said, "I told *you* that," and he answered, "Here's what we are going to do for it. For the pain, we are going to give you a pain killer. For the muscle spasms, we are going to give you a muscle relaxer. And for the swelling, we are going to give you an anti-inflammatory."

That made sense to me so I took the medication and fortunately for me they did NOT work. Two weeks later, I was still sick and nauseous from the medication. I wasn't back wrestling yet and my mom was alert enough to recommend we seek a different solution and brought me to the chiropractor.

The chiropractor evaluated me, laid me on a table, adjusted my neck, and I was instantly 90 percent better. At that time, I didn't understand this was a "different" kind of doctor. I asked him what he'd just done and he explained how the physical stress from what I did created in my neck what he referred to as subluxation or mal-alignment of the segments in my spine that was irritating nerves.

He said that he introduced a force into my neck — an adjustment — to help align my spine to reduce the strain on my nervous system. I deduced that was the reason I felt better instantly and asked him, "Why didn't anyone else do this?" He told me it was because they have a different philosophy about health care. I went back for a series of adjustments and asked many more questions. One day, the chiropractor took a good amount of time over his lunch to explain the whole philosophy of chiropractic to me and it was at that point I decided it was what I wanted to do with my life.

Where do you currently reside and how are you spending your time these days?

I reside in Mahwah, New Jersey and I spend my time running two companies. One is the Chiropractic Leadership Alliance, which has about 8,000 clients on six continents. We also developed breakthrough technology for chiropractors to help them better assess their patients, quantify neurological function and neurospinal health.

In line with that, we also do a lot of educational work, seminars, our "On Purpose" audio program, and interviews with the prominent minds of the health care world.

We also have Creating Wellness Alliance chiropractic-based lifestyle wellness centers. Right now, we have about 300 Creating Wellness Centers, most of which are in North America although we also have them in New Zealand, Ireland, and the United Kingdom.

We have developed technology for them so they can quantify lifestyle wellness and create lifestyle recommendations that incorporate an entire lifestyle program for an individual. People improve their general health and wellness status as they're getting their chiropractic adjustments. We're building a national and international "brand" of chiropractic in the context of wellness that adjusts consumers' concept of chiropractic. It goes from being back pain oriented to lifestyle wellness oriented. That is what the essential core of chiropractic is.

How does the profession differ now from when you first became involved?

I got out of chiropractic school in 1983, so we are looking at many years. The profession changed in many ways but in others ways, it hasn't changed at all. Dr. Christopher Kent was reading an old newsletter from a chiropractic association in New York recently and he commented to me, "All you have to do is change the date and everything else applies." The publication was from the 1930s and the articles focused on various issues chiropractic was tackling back then such as the debates raging within the profession and the political landscape where medicine had the authority in health care and chiropractic was trying to define its identity and distinctions. A lot of the same rhetoric is here today.

The first significant change is the Internet; it's changed everything. When I got out of school it was almost impossible, as a consumer, to find out anything about chiropractic. As a senior, I tried to find information in libraries, bookstores, and health food stores but I could find nothing on chiropractic. There was no Internet back then and people didn't have personal computers. To find out anything about chiropractic you had to find a chiropractor. It was very difficult.

The playing field has leveled a lot with the advent of the Internet and web searching. You can Google "chiropractic" and be reading for the rest of your life. That's one profound equalizer. On your computer screen the big drug company ads are no bigger than they are for an individual chiropractor. The ability to communicate the chiropractic philosophy and explain what chiropractic practice is to the community at large is phenomenal.

The second difference is that, during the past two years there's been more positive press on chiropractic than I think I've ever seen. The mass media is starting to come our way and a big part of that is the wellness revolution. As I mentioned, when I got out of school there was no talk about wellness, health clubs, health foods, or bottled water. In 1990, wellness was barely a blip on the screen of economics and now it's a $500 billion industry — more than half a trillion dollars and growing.

Lifestyle wellness, which is a much popularized thing in the culture today that wasn't there before, is aligned closely with the principles of chiropractic. Further, we're starting to see many celebrities speak out publicly about how chiropractic helped them. Jerry Rice, the famed football player, just became the spokesperson for the Foundation for Chiropractic Progress. Madonna announced her world tour and talked about her chiropractor. Lance Armstrong and his chiropractor make public proclamations. You see our chiropractic Insight evaluation equipment in the locker rooms at a number of professional sports arenas.

Suddenly, we're seeing an explosion of chiropractic utilization in high-profile areas and it's trickling down into the general public. The consumer is starting to hear more about chiropractic and getting more excited about engaging in chiropractic.

How do chiropractic and performance relate?

Chiropractic and performance are inextricably related. Chiropractic deals with the nervous system and the mind-body connection. When you have stress — which comes in three dimensions, physical, biochemical, and psychological — that is beyond what your body can normally adapt to and dissipate, there's compromise in function and performance. The subluxation is a sign that individual stress is beyond the person's general adaptive potential, not to the point of death but to the point he or she can't fully function. This will lead to compromise in nervous system function and that translates into tension patterns that will change the alignment of spinal segments.

Suddenly, we're seeing an explosion of chiropractic utilization in high-profile areas and it's trickling down into the general public. The consumer is starting to hear more about chiropractic and getting more excited about engaging in chiropractic.

When people are in a state of subluxation, they are holding these patterns, their bodies are in a defensive physiology, and therefore don't grow and perform nearly as well as they could. When we identify these patterns of subluxation, which are compromising health performance, we can apply a constructive force — what we call an adjustment — to release them. Now, the person is running at higher capacity. We're basically upgrading efficiency and function; therefore the individual will perform better.

This is why athletes, for example, do so much better with chiropractic. Most of them know it's not a matter of getting rid of back or neck pain. Chiropractic allows them to perform better, gives them longevity on the field, improves their reflexes and eye-hand coordination, allows them to run faster, and jump higher. When you start tuning up the nervous system, you tune up everything because the nerve system is the master system in control of the body. When you start to have an impact on neural processing and efficiency of neural processing, you affect overall performance.

How does chiropractic relate to a person realizing his or her fullest human potential?

I think the answer is pretty much everything I just said. We live our lives through our nervous system and if we're trying to actualize full potential, trying to expand our capacities and expression of life, we're going to be limited by the efficiency of our neural function and processing. The beneficial impact that chiropractic has (and incidentally what the technology of the Insight equipment measures and demonstrates) translates into an enhanced and fuller life.

How does chiropractic offer people an opportunity to realize an enhanced quality of life?

Enhanced quality of life depends not only on the chiropractic adjustment but on the chiropractic lifestyle. If you live with too much stress in your life and don't modify your lifestyle to reduce these negative stressors, you can keep getting adjusted but you don't really progress very well. It's critical that we live healthier in the physical, bio-chemical, and psychological dimensions while we get adjusted. Then we can have transformation of our individual experience of the expression of life.

What do you feel has happened to the chiropractic profession that may have limited it from being seen by the world in its true nature?

First, the American Medical Association (AMA) conspired to destroy the chiropractic profession. It's well documented and has been adjudicated in courts of law where it was determined that the AMA and affiliated organizations were in violation of U.S. anti-trust laws and conspired to eliminate the chiropractic profession. That had a major negative impact on the perception of chiropractic. I don't think there is any doubt about it.

Second, many of the edicts of the Council on Chiropractic Education have taken chiropractic education away from its core philosophy, core principles, and moved it toward a more allopathic model. Much of the education, testing, and national boards, etc. are virtually allopathic slanted. That's created an identity crisis to a large extent within the profession. Students graduating and going out into the field are confused about what it means to be a chiropractor.

We have this unique principle that is brilliant and powerful and when practiced has phenomenal impact and results. It's been diluted and confused with more allopathic medical principles and as a result practitioners have lost their focus.

I'd like to be crystal clear here. I am not saying that medicine is something bad or inferior. Quite the opposite. I would not want to live in a culture that didn't have medical services available. However, it's something that I would refer to as sick care crisis intervention — not health care. When you confuse sick care with health care or take sick care and try to pass it off as health care, you end up with a sick culture, which is why we have a problem in society today. No amount of money will solve that problem.

If you are trying to simultaneously practice sick care and promote healthy wellness ideals, you end up wondering who the heck you are and the practice gets confused.

Third, to be a chiropractor means (more so years ago than now) to be a rebel and not part of the mainstream. The only type of person who would want to engage in such would be someone who is an individual thinker. This profession was built on rugged individualists and rugged individualism.

Having a bunch of strong-willed individuals grouped together in a common profession, each with our own ideas about things, challenges our ability to create a unified message that resonates well in the culture.

Chiropractic has become tagged as a pain relief specialty. In your opinion what more does it have to offer people?

Obviously, chiropractic offers individuals much more than back and neck pain relief. It offers them the opportunity to express and experience a greater life in total. I said earlier that you live your life through your nervous system and that nothing happens within the realm of the human experience that doesn't involve neural function. By improving the efficiency of neural function, by taking the body out of defense physiology and toward growth, the impact of chiropractic is as vast as the experience of life itself.

I consider chiropractic to be so powerful that it can't be limited to what some might consider health care. It affects your entire life. So many people are so overstressed they can't sleep at night without a pill. Before long, instead of having a sleeping problem they have a pill problem. There are people who feel great anxiety about the economy. Instead of dealing with the anxiety, they take a psychiatric drug, which numbs them to the anxiety. They're also trading one type of problem for another. The pills that they're taking to solve their problems aren't vitamins but serious chemicals that alter their human existence.

What chiropractic offers people is a way to contend with the stress of life naturally. It allows the body to process, heal, grow, and experience wellness from the inside out, rather than drugging it and forcing it into altered states of physiology through medication. I'm not saying that medication is never necessary but I am saying it should only be utilized in crisis situations. Medicine is not a lifestyle. People think they can eat poorly and just take pills to lower their cholesterol and that solves their problem. Nothing is further from the truth.

What is the purpose of the chiropractic adjustment and how does not receiving chiropractic care impact one's life?

> **What chiropractic offers people is a way to contend with the stress of life naturally. It allows the body to process, heal, grow, and experience wellness from the inside out, rather than drugging it and forcing it into altered states of physiology through medication.**

I gave a presentation to a room of chiropractors last weekend and asked them to do a thought experiment with me. I said, "I want you all to think about the last chiropractic adjustment you received." I then told them, "Now imagine that was the *last* chiropractic adjustment you would receive for the rest of your life."

It was interesting because you could see how the entire room just freaked out. It would be inconceivable for them to go the rest of their lives without being adjusted.

Then I said, "Now, I would like you to consider your life and ask yourself where you would be right now if you had never received a chiropractic adjustment." Again, it was shocking to them to even consider how their lives would have been if they had never been adjusted.

I was making the point that the majority of people who live in our culture have either never had a chiropractic adjustment or will never be adjusted for the rest of their lives. That is a pretty horrible scenario when you know what chiropractic is and you have experienced its benefits.

For me, my family, and my loved ones, not being checked and adjusted through chiropractic could never be a consideration. I don't want to live in mediocrity or just survive and get through it. For me, having an extraordinary life and therefore receiving chiropractic is vital. The purpose of the chiropractic adjustment specifically is to release patterns of subluxation so the nervous system can express and operate on a more efficient level. As a result, we experience better health and well-being.

What is your favorite quote and how has it impacted your life?

I don't know if I have a single favorite quote. Since we're talking about chiropractic, two quotes come to mind that I believe are important and related to each other. The first is from Aristotle: "Nature does nothing uselessly." It's very important to understand that in order to be a health care provider. A derivative quote is from Ayn Rand, who said, "In order for nature to be commanded, it must be obeyed." I found that to be a very powerful quote in the context of what we are talking about here with health care.

How is chiropractic unique and what does it offer that other health professions do not?

Chiropractic has a unique philosophy and the basis of that philosophy is vitalism — that biological organisms are not machines. I was interviewing the great surgeon Bernie Siegel for our "On Purpose" series and he told me that one of the questions on the application for medical school was, "Why do you want to become a medical doctor?" The most common answer was, "I always had an interest in the human body." Whenever he saw that response, he'd tell the applicant, "Well, you better remember a *person* comes inside that body."

That is essentially what vitalism is about and that's what chiropractic is about. It's about life, the experience, and the expression of life. It's not just fixing a bad part. That really isn't the foundational intention of chiropractic. The foundational intention of chiropractic is to allow the body to heal more efficiently and express life on a higher level.

What do you sense was the intention behind the creation of chiropractic?

The intention behind the creation of chiropractic was to bring to the world a healing discipline that would solve many of humanity's problems and help humanity transcend certain limitations that existed in the culture and the environment. It was — and still is — a very big idea and vision. Its beauty is its simplicity. It's not hard to give chiropractic care or to receive it. As a result, there is this simple thing that one human being can do to help and support another that changes the entire path that person is on, for the better.

Who are some of your mentors and what impact have they had on your life?

I have to start with my mom especially and my dad for owning a health food store and being different from everybody else. That was back before it was popular. Also, my mom was a thinker and encouraged me to get chiropractic care. I've learned a lot from my mom about positive thinking and empowerment that's helped me achieve much in life.

In chiropractic, Christopher Kent is certainly, perhaps more than any other individual, the one who has had the most profound impact on my thinking and understanding. Fred Barge and Ian Grassam were both great mentors. Sid Williams certainly had a big impact when I was at Life Chiropractic College. Guy Riekeman is a great chiropractic leader and a good friend of mine. Fabrizio Mancini is one of my dearest friends in the world. Gerry Clum was an instructor when I was a chiropractic student and he had a profound impact on me. Economist Paul Zane Pilzer, who wrote "The Wellness Revolution," is another mentor. There are definitely many more than that and I don't want to leave anyone out.

What turns you on creatively, spiritually, or emotionally?

At the risk of sounding simplistic, life!

Where do you see the profession 10 years from now?

In 10 years, chiropractic will be in a better and yet a more challenging position. The entire third-party pay model is going to be transformed within the next decade. It could be transformed in one of two ways.

Health care could be socialized (if it is, the best thing for chiropractic is to be left out of that system). If the health care system is not socialized, we'll end up more toward a free market system, which will be very good for chiropractic. That's where health savings accounts and health reimbursement arrangements will take over the marketplace and instead of an employer-driven health care system we'll have a consumer-driven health care system.

It's going to tip one way or the other but one thing I know for sure is that what's going on right now is going to end. That being the case, there will be a lot of purging of the profession. Many people in this profession who have been on a diet of insurance may end up no longer having a career. It's sad but it's coming. I already saw one wave of it with HMOs coming in. I saw another wave with modifications in workers compensation and personal injury. Every time those changes occur, there are chiropractors who end up going by the wayside.

In line with this there's also going to be a big move culturally toward more proactive behaviors in health care. That's chiropractic's huge opportunity and it needs to get to that marketplace with the right message and attract these people. Ten years from now one possible outcome is increased chiropractic utilization by people coming for the right reasons and chiropractic giving up its insurance dependency. That is certainly what I am working for.

What profession other than your own would you like to have attempted?

Chiropractic is always where I wanted to be and the view of my career is entirely new, different, and changing all of the time. I'm not in practice right now but I am in the practice of business within chiropractic and health care.

Are there any other comments you'd like to share about the wonders of chiropractic?

The wonders of chiropractic are so extraordinary and profound that an individual can spend a lifetime trying to fully understanding them. The implications keep running deeper, and the deeper you get, the more you start to realize on a practical level how profound a solution chiropractic is for many of the challenges facing the world right now. Chiropractic extends well beyond the construct of what most people would consider health care; it's much more connected to what it is to live a fuller and more actualized life. It's sad when chiropractic patients never get the opportunity to find out the full breadth and implications of chiropractic. What's even sadder is when chiropractors don't get it either.

Years from now when people look at your tombstone, what would you want them to read?

I already know what that is. The tombstone reads:
"Here lies Patrick Gentempo, Jr., who was disliked by some but loved by more as he challenged the hearts and minds of the mediocre while he improved the world in a significant way."

I don't know if they'll let me bring it to my office but I'm going to have my tombstone carved and I'm going to look at it every day. If I don't know the statement of my life now, I don't want others to figure it out after I'm dead.

და

Patrick Gentempo, Jr., D.C., is co-founder and CEO of the Chiropractic Leadership Alliance. He is an internationally renowned lecturer, researcher, and chiropractic business consultant. As one of the largest draws in chiropractic today, he is famous for his ability to integrate the philosophy, science, clinical practice, and business of chiropractic without contradiction.

Along with Dr. Christopher Kent, he co-developed the Total Solution Program, Insight Millennium Subluxation Station, the On Purpose monthly audio subscription service and "Celebrity Marketing Program," a powerful consumer marketing and education package for the chiropractor.

An accomplished entrepreneur and wellness expert, Dr. Gentempo announced the launch of his newest company, the Creating Wellness Alliance (CWA), in January 2003. CWA is the result of six years of exhaustive observation and intensive research by Dr. Gentempo to create a national, then international, brand of chiropractic in the context of wellness. His vision for Creating Wellness has attracted media giant William Shatner as its celebrity spokesperson, and is destined to position the chiropractic profession as the leader of the wellness revolution.

The teacher who is indeed wise does not bid you to enter the house of his wisdom but rather leads you to the threshold of your mind.

Khalil Gibran

Reggie Gold

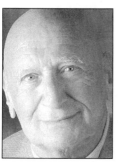

I want to start by saying I don't act in the same ways that B.J. would have acted. I think chiropractic has come a long way since then. You must understand that I don't hold true to the original ideas.

Where are you from originally and what was your childhood like?

I was raised in the slums of London. My childhood was just a childhood and I don't remember much about it.

What inspired you to get involved with chiropractic?

Chiropractic was the first thing that ever made sense to me. I had been bothered with hay fever and asthma all my life. I went to the medical doctors and the answers they gave didn't satisfy me. I asked them, "Why do I have hay fever? Why me and not my brothers or my parents? Why only me?" The answer I got was, "You're the unlucky one I guess."

I just could not accept that hay fever was the result of bad luck; there had to be some other cause. Eventually, somebody told me about chiropractic. I went down to talk to this chiropractor and he explained that it was not associated with luck at all. Something physically was causing it. I asked what that was and he said that he didn't know yet. He said it was obvious that my body wasn't performing properly and that it was his job to find out why. He said it was possible that this thing called a subluxation was causing my body to malfunction.

That was the first time I had heard that there could be a physical cause to explain why I had the hay fever and my brothers and sisters didn't. That kind of answer made sense to me and he further explained about subluxation and nerve interference. Long before I experienced any chance of success or not, I enrolled in Palmer College in 1954.

Where do you currently reside and how are you spending your time these days?

I currently reside in Bala Cynwyd, Pennsylvania, just outside Philadelphia, and I spend most of my time lecturing and teaching. I spend my time trying to change chiropractors' attitudes and trying to change the mindset they learned in school. I feel that chiropractors come into chiropractic with so much baggage that they are too rigid and inflexible. They come in with certain fixed ideas picked up from medical propaganda and I spend my time traveling the world attempting to shift their mindset as to what chiropractic truly is. I've spent my life trying to change chiropractors away from the treatment of disease into what I feel they should have been doing in the first place and that is correcting vertebral subluxations whether anybody has a disease or not.

How does the profession differ now from when you first became involved?

How does it differ? Well, I changed it! I graduated Palmer in 1957 and went out practicing the way B.J. told me. I heard people saying that chiropractic got sick people well and I initially went out to try and cure people's sickness. That is the farthest thing from my mind now. I have no interest in sickness, no interest in disease, or even in health. I think chiropractic's biggest mistake was to get involved in the health profession in the first place. That was B.J.'s major error and he passed it on to me and every other chiropractor.

Everybody has been under the impression that chiropractic is supposed to cure disease, chiropractic gets sick people well, the power that made the body heals the body, etc., etc. — and that is simply not true. If you follow the philosophy of chiropractic, it has nothing to do with health and sickness at all. It has nothing to do with sick people getting well. I created a new vision of chiropractic, one that made total sense to me.

How do chiropractic and performance relate?

Chiropractic is all about performance. I started out thinking that it was only about health performance and that the body's job is to protect itself from disease, that we have a built-in immune system, and that subluxation causes the immune system to function imperfectly.

When I further analyzed that concept, I realized that subluxation causes all functions to perform imperfectly. If you have nerve interference, nothing you do, say, or think remains unaffected. You can't do anything at your best as long as you have the subluxation. My job is to get chiropractors to realize this and concentrate on the correction of subluxation whether people are sick or not. If they have subluxation, any performance is reduced and interfered with.

How does chiropractic relate to a person realizing his or her fullest human potential?

Again, it's the same thing. As long as there is nerve interference, the body can't live up to its potential. Every function of human life — mental, physical, spiritual, and intellectual, every function of the human body — is impaired by subluxation. So when you have a subluxation, your driving is involved and affected to the extent you cannot drive properly or safely. You cannot coordinate, you cannot balance, and you cannot harmonize your activities. You cannot think as clearly, your moods are affected, and every function in life is negatively affected by subluxation.

How does chiropractic offer people an opportunity to realize an enhanced quality of life?

It doesn't really enhance the quality. The maximum quality of performance is already built in and subluxation interferes with that. Correction of subluxation allows the body a better chance of functioning normally, whatever *normal* may be for that person. Sometimes the only result of getting rid of your subluxation is that you will live two years longer.

What do you feel has happened to the chiropractic profession that may have limited it from being seen by the world in its true nature.

It was never presented to the world in its true nature. Chiropractic didn't make a mistake somewhere along the line. Chiropractic made its mistake on day one! In fact, the day before there was chiropractic, D.D. Palmer was trying to cure disease with magnetic healing. When he discovered the chiropractic principle, it was just another treatment and another way of treating disease. In other words, before chiropractic had even gotten started it had already gone wrong because D.D. Palmer produced a method of treating disease without drugs.

In fact, the way D.D. Palmer saw it, chiropractic was a part of the practice of medicine. The treatment of disease, if you look it up in the dictionary, is defined as the practice of medicine utilizing any method of treating and curing disease. If chiropractic diagnoses, treats, or cures disease, it is part of medicine. We went wrong before we ever started as a profession.

Unfortunately, there is no chiropractic school in existence today that teaches the truth about chiropractic. In fact, most chiropractors wouldn't attend such a school if it did exist. We come into chiropractic with a lot of baggage that stops us from learning about real chiropractic and the truth. Then we get to school and pick up more negative baggage and medical thinking.

How did you come up with reframing chiropractic and how did it come to you what chiropractic was truly about?

It was there for anybody who wanted it. I just happened to see it first. I was thinking about it and I asked myself questions. Why do some people get rid of their backaches with chiropractic care and other people don't? I realized the claims we were making about chiropractic were totally wrong. Chiropractic does not cure disease and it is not meant to cure disease. Chiropractic allows the body to function at a higher level.

Chiropractic has become tagged as a pain relief specialty. In your opinion, what more does it have to offer?

I think the relief of pain and the ability of the body to repair or cure itself of disease represents about five percent of chiropractic. The other 95 percent has nothing to do with pain or disease. The body just functions better. People treat their kids better when they're not subluxated. I wonder how many battered wives and battered children there are because of subluxation. Yet, we don't offer chiropractic as prevention of maltreatment of kids. We don't offer chiropractic as a way of driving a car better or driving a golf ball better.

Every function of life is affected by subluxation and chiropractic will never get to its rightful place until chiropractors themselves realize this. We have to get away from the image of chiropractic getting sick people well; get away from talking about sickness and disease. We have to tell people the real truth of chiropractic, that if you have a vertebral subluxation, you are better off without it always and under every circumstance. There is never a time that a subluxation does not do harm. Looking only at symptoms and disease is ridiculous and misses 95 percent of the damage done by subluxation.

We have to therefore change the mindset of chiropractors. Chiropractors are being bombarded constantly with the attempts to cure disease. They are not focusing on anything else and therefore they are totally missing the point of chiropractic. Chiropractic has become a part of medicine.

What is the purpose of the chiropractic adjustment and how does not receiving chiropractic care impact one's life?

First of all, the chiropractic adjustment is not a chiropractic adjustment. Chiropractors do not adjust bones and we don't give an adjustment. We can't set the bone back where it belongs simply because we don't know where it belongs. That is a secret known only to the body itself. The innate wisdom of the body knows its own subluxations and knows the position the bone must be restored to in order to correct the subluxation. Only the Innate Intelligence has the ability to adjust. It's really wrong to call it a *chiropractic* adjustment.

Far more adjustments are given by accident than are ever given intentionally by chiropractors. Whether an adjustment is given through an intentional force or through an accidental force makes no difference at all. If the subluxation is gone, it's gone. If it hasn't gone, then it's still there.

Chiropractors have been raised to look at the few symptoms they can see and think that's the whole picture. In other words, we're thinking medically.

How does it impact the world at large? Most subluxations are left there because we have no method of recognizing them. We tend to look for the effects of a subluxation or the results of an adjustment. We do not have the methodology to find out what damage has been done to a psyche or a physical body. Chiropractors have been raised to look at the few symptoms they can see and think that's the whole picture. In other words, we're thinking medically.

We need to improve our methodology of locating and identifying vertebral subluxation. Then we need to improve our mindset so when we've introduced a force, we can post-check and make sure the subluxation is gone. Right now we have no methodology. Chiropractic has a long way to go in changing its methodology to find ways of determining the presence or absence of subluxation. Right now we can only go by symptoms and thousands of subluxations have no symptoms.

It's not a subluxation unless it involves nerve interference. You can't actually measure it but you get certain information that leads you to a conclusion. You then tally up the total of the evidence and you go by the weight of evidence. The Vertebraille Method I developed measures what the body is trying to change. I have a theory that if the body is trying to change it, it should be changed. I palpate the muscles that move the bones and follow the body's direction. What bone are those muscles trying to move, and in which direction? The body certainly knows how far to move it. I have total trust in the Innate Intelligence in the body.

If we don't call it the chiropractic adjustment, what should we call it instead?

Just the adjustment. I think we'd be a lot better if we'd refer to it as "The Innate Adjustment" because only the Innate Intelligence knows whether it's an adjustment or not. When you put a force into somebody's spine, you don't really know whether the bone has gone back into place or not. There is an innate awareness of every innate need so the body knows whether it's subluxated or not.

Please share with us what Innate Intelligence is to you.

Innate Intelligence, I would say, is that part of Universal Intelligence or that expression of Universal Intelligence, which exists within every living creature in order to nurture and protect it. That is what we call the Innate Intelligence, the inborn wisdom of the body.

Roughly three hundred and fifty years ago a great physiologist referred to it as the "Wisdom of the Body," and that term is perfectly as good today as it was then. We don't need terms like Innate Intelligence as long as we understand that there is some indefinable force within every living thing that maintains life. Particularly in human beings, it functions by the intellectual expression of the brain operating through the nerve system to reach all parts of the body. In a tree, there is no nerve system and yet the tree still functions the same way to protect itself. The trouble is that we have invented a pretense — Innate Intelligence. We talk about it as though "You have an Innate Intelligence." That is not really the truth. The truth is an Innate Intelligence has you. Innate Intelligence is Universal Intelligence expressing within you.

What is your favorite quote and how has it impacted your life?

I don't think there is a favorite. You can use, "You have to be a little cracked, that's what lets the light in." That's an original and you're getting it right from the source.

How is chiropractic unique and what does it offer that other health professions do not?

Number one, chiropractic is **not** a health profession. That is the big mistake that chiropractors have made and that is why chiropractic is not on the map. They have tried to make it a health profession. Chiropractic is only interested in correcting subluxation. Affecting the health is maybe only five percent of that. The other 95 percent has nothing to do with health. If chiropractors would mention subluxation and not talk about health, they would solve their own problems. All of their problems arise from linking chiropractic with health.

A subluxation messes up the entire body. True, it messes up your health but it messes up everything else too. By focusing on health, we have made an enemy of the medical profession — which they never should have been — and we have limited ourselves into a tiny fraction of the real purpose of getting people free from subluxation. The whole idea is, when you have a vertebral subluxation everything in your life goes wrong and it will never be corrected until the subluxation is corrected.

If we can teach the public about what chiropractic is, they will force the chiropractors to do the right thing. How do you get the true message of chiropractic across without the chiropractor as the intermediary? It's a double task and I think it starts with changing a few chiropractors.

What do you sense was the intention behind the creation of chiropractic?

The original intent was to cure disease. If D.D. Palmer had any other notion, we have no indication of that. He always talked about curing disease. The first adjustment was given to cure Harvey Lillard's deafness and every other adjustment since then by him and by his son was given to cure something. Even the *prevention* of disease was not mentioned, it was the *curing* of disease.

The first realization in my practice was that instead of curing disease we'd do much better to try and prevent disease. From there, I went into the understanding that the subluxation doesn't just mess up your health, it messes up your entire life. It disturbs your balance, your emotions, and your spiritual values. Everything is coordinated by the nerves from the brain. When that communication between the brain and the tissue cell is altered in any way, the result is a disharmony of the entire body and a lessened potential of every function.

In your opinion, what needs to be changed in chiropractic, and when it is changed, what will chiropractic look like?

First of all, I don't know that it can be changed. We've developed tests to qualify people to be chiropractors. They are medical tests and not chiropractic in nature whatsoever. Every chiropractor is trained to think medically. How do you change them from that into accepting the idea of what chiropractic should be? I don't know. I don't know how to get through to the chiropractors. That has been my entire life mission.

In my life, 50 years of work has produced maybe 15-20 chiropractors who finally got the big idea. That is after teaching and lecturing to millions. Even those who I thought got the big idea still explain chiropractic in terms of health and sickness. As long as the chiropractor talks health and sickness, the public can never get the big idea of what chiropractic is all about. Chiropractic is much bigger than health and sickness. If I ask a chiropractor what health means, he or she will say health includes everything else about the body. The public hears the words "health" and "disease" and they don't think of everything else about the body, they just think of the things that the medical profession deals with.

This is why I say that the only hope for chiropractic in the future is to divorce itself from that medical image. We need a lot of hard-nosed chiropractors who really understand the big idea and are prepared to work on changing the world's opinion of chiropractic. That's very difficult to do when all of the baggage they take into chiropractic in the first place is reinforced by their medical education. You cannot become a licensed chiropractor without that medical education. We have kind of sealed our own fate. We've agreed to practice medicine and do what they tell us. They have said, "Okay, you can deal with backaches and headaches. All other disease has to be referred to the medical people." We have played their game.

Who are some of your mentors and what impact have they had on your life?

I don't know that I've had any mentors. These ideas originated with me.

What are some things, if any, you had to give up in order to devote your life to chiropractic?

I don't think I have given up anything. I've gained a sense of mission. I finally found something I can truly believe in. I don't have to lie about it and it has become my whole life. In other words chiropractic has given me a purpose for living.

What turns you on creatively, spiritually, or emotionally?

Just the realization that chiropractic, as I had learned it, didn't make any bloody sense. The pretense that the only reason for being sick is because you're subluxated is simply not true. There are lots of reasons you could be sick. Let's say it's genetic and you inherited certain things. All the adjustments in the world are not going to change that in your generation. I think there's a built-in limitation to the human body and the limitation varies from person to person in the same way that everything else varies from person to person.

Where do you see the profession 10 years from now?

Just as mixed up and confused as it is right now! I don't see chiropractic under that name becoming any better than it is already. The only hope for chiropractic lies in the hands of the spinologists. By virtue of their training and the laws, they're not allowed to practice medicine. They do exactly what a chiropractor does except they are not allowed, by law, to talk about it in terms of health and sickness. I think our entire future lies in the hands of others.

> **We have already screwed up the world so much, as far as chiropractic is concerned. As B.J. said, "Chiropractic will probably disappear and appear again under another name.**

We have already screwed up the world so much, as far as chiropractic is concerned. As B.J. said, "Chiropractic will probably disappear and appear again under another name." I really think that was the truth. I sincerely believe that spinology might well be the answer. The only three schools I know of for this are in Australia, Spain, and Ireland. The biggest one is in Spain and that was created by a graduate spinologist of mine, who studied in Philadelphia and trained the others. He's been running the school in Spain for the last 30 years. It started off in Valencia and has recently moved its headquarters to Madrid.

A fellow from Ireland, who I trained as a chiropractor, decided — as a result of my talks with him — that he really didn't want to be a chiropractor. He went to Australia to learn spinology but was unhappy with the director of that school so he talked to the people in Spain and they sent him to Ireland. He went to practice in Ireland and since then has started a school and is teaching there as well.

Spinology is true chiropractic and by law they're not permitted to practice a healing art. They're not trained in medicine and therefore cannot practice medicine. Chiropractors are trained in medicine and are allowed to practice limited medicine by utilizing manipulative therapy.

The only hope for the future of chiropractic lies with non-chiropractors. We need to take all of the chiropractors with good potential and redirect them into spinology. Certainly the philosophy of spinology makes a whole lot more sense than the distorted chiropractic philosophy.

What profession other than your own would you like to have attempted?

None. I had to learn chiropractic and deduce from it the next direction.

Please share with us the concept of a "box on the wall."

A box on the wall can still work today and is the purest form of chiropractic. It allows chiropractors to do their job with total freedom and money is not a factor at all. If people put nothing in the box, they still receive the same benefit from getting rid of the subluxation. A past chiropractic college president and others have said that if we don't charge enough money, people won't get well. That's absolute nonsense. We explain to the people that their financial situation is none of our business and we trust them to know what to do.

I advise people, after their subluxations are brought under control, to come in for the rest of their lives for regular care once a week to have their spines checked.

Look at it this way, there's no *right* price for a chiropractic adjustment. Let's say we're dealing with an architect married to an accountant. Maybe they're earning a quarter of a million dollars a year and have no kids. How much can they afford to pay each time they come in?

I advise people, after their subluxations are brought under control, to come in for the rest of their lives for regular care once a week to have their spines checked. In the situation above, the husband and wife are both professionals and they earn good money. How much should they pay per visit?

In California right now, the average fee is $55 per person. In other parts of the country it may be a little less or a little more. Alaska and Hawaii are more but generally I think that between $40 and $50 is the average. West Virginia and Mississippi may be less. Forty dollars is a generous fee for the architect who, with his wife, is pulling in a quarter of a million a year, with no kids to take care of.

Now let's change the situation. We have a single mother with five kids. What should she pay? She has the same subluxation doing the same damage to her life. How much is an adjustment worth to her? Whatever we charge is too much for some people and too little for others. So, let them determine their own fee according to their means.

In other words, there is no correct fee. This is what got me out of the fee system and into the box-on-the-wall system that chiropractors use today around the country. Since there is no proper fee, the chiropractor ought to put a box on the wall and allow people to determine their own fee. I have touched a lot of lives with my suggestion that a box on the wall is a wonderful way to go. Some of the wealthiest chiropractors practice that way and some of the best donors to the colleges and other funds are box-on-the-wall chiropractors.

Some worry that people will rip you off practicing that way or that some won't put money in at all because you don't see what goes in. That's true, some people will rip you off, but then some people will rip you off no matter what you do. If we charge insurance companies and then the insurance company refuses to pay for some reason, what do we do? Go after the patients themselves? With a box on the wall you're totally free from all that crap.

Are there any other comments you'd like to share about the wonders of chiropractic?

The wonders of chiropractic are so simple that they're almost not worth discussing. You could discuss the whole thing in one sentence. The correction of subluxation allows the body to work at full potential, in the same way that the subluxation, by its very presence, inhibits the function of the body. The big idea in chiropractic is that if you have a subluxation you'd be better off without it and that just flies over every chiropractor's head.

I explain it to the public in terms of body chemistry. Performance is always directed and controlled by body chemistry. If your chemistry is normal under the body's own innate control, then the functions of the body are as perfect as they are ever going to get. Body chemistry is controlled by the billions of cells that make the chemicals. The cells that make the chemicals are controlled by the nerve system and the nerves are protected by bone. A subluxation develops. That causes one of the two problems humanity has. Or as B.J. put it, there are only two diseases: too much and too little. You either have too much of this chemical or too little of that one. If the chemicals are perfect and under the brain's control, then the body functions at its own maximum potential. Not necessarily perfection, but the best it's capable of doing.

Chiropractic's role should be to bring about the correction of subluxation. Actually, the chiropractor doesn't adjust but introduces a force intelligently contrived in the hope that the body will then be able to adapt that force into an adjustment. The body alone knows where the bone belongs.

The philosophy of chiropractic is so bloody simple. The problem is that it's too simple for most chiropractors to understand. Most chiropractors think that it has to be complicated and they think there's a lot to learn. There's almost nothing to learn. You should be able to train a chiropractor in six months from a zero point out of high school to be able to find the subluxation and introduce the force whereby the body can correct the subluxation.

Years from now when people look at your tombstone, what would you want them to read?

I think my original epigram is the one I still live which is, "If you are not out to change the world, your whole life is just a waste of time."

Reggie Gold, D.C., Ph.C., graduated Summa Cum Laude as class valedictorian from Palmer College in 1957, and has served in various capacities in state and national organizations ever since. He founded one chiropractic college, assisted in the founding of another, taught philosophy at three colleges, and has lectured at most of the others. In addition, he's lectured about chiropractic at several medical schools, represented chiropractic on radio and television, testified before state legislatures and foreign governments, and started free chiropractic training for the Quechua Indians on the High Andes Mountains of Peru.

Dr. Gold has received hundreds of honors including the prestigious "International Humanitarian Award" from the World Congress of Chiropractic. He earned a PhC degree from Palmer College and a Doctorate in Humanities (honoris causa) from Sherman College, is a distinguished Fellow of the International Chiropractors Association, and a member of the Palmer Academy.

On top of all this, he managed to run one of the most successful practices ever — known at a time and in a place where the practice of chiropractic was illegal!

Christopher Kent

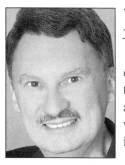

Where are you from originally and what was your childhood like?

I'm originally from Milwaukee and I was one of those fortunate people who got into chiropractic relatively early in life. As a child, I guess I had a pretty normal life. I was fortunate in that there was minimal medical intervention and I became interested in chiropractic when I was 16.

I wondered what chiropractic was and I asked my mother, who worked at the medical college. Her reply was, "That's someone who cracks your bones." My response to her was, "Cracks your bones? You mean they fracture?" She said, "I guess they must because you can hear them snap." I said, "Why would anyone want that done?" and she said, "I don't know, I certainly wouldn't."

My best friend at the time, who was rational and seemingly ambulatory, was talking about how wonderful chiropractic was yet my mother was planting the seed of iatrogenic fractures. I came up with what I *thought* was a clever plan. I called a chiropractor and asked him if I could do an interview because I was doing a report for school. I asked him what we all have asked so many times, "What is it that chiropractors do?"

His response was very simple. "Chiropractic is based on four simple concepts," he explained. "The first is that the body is a self-healing organism. Cut your finger and it heals. Cut the finger of a corpse and it doesn't. Life is what heals. Second, the nervous system is the master system of the body and every aspect of the human experience is processed through the nervous system. Three, when there is interference with the function of the nervous system, not only can it compromise your physical well-being, but because it distorts your perception of the world and inhibits your ability to respond to the world, it can lead to psycho-emotional issues as well. When this happens to a significant number of people in a society, you have a sick society."

Finally, he said, "What I do as a chiropractor is locate and correct the cause of that interference." The rest, as they say, is history. Not long after I became a patient he said, "I think you should become a chiropractor." It made perfect sense, so I did.

Where did you attend chiropractic college and when?

I went to Palmer and graduated in 1973. It was a great time and the place was very alive. Chiropractic was very much integrated into the basic sciences and there was an especially strong culture and feeling of family.

Where do you currently reside and how are you spending your time these days?

I am currently living in Ramsey, New Jersey. I am co-founder, with Patrick Gentempo, of the Chiropractic Leadership Alliance. I work doing a number of things. I prepare the material for our audio service subscription programs known as "On Purpose." Another thing I work on is the technical development of our chiropractic instrumentation, the Subluxation Station. I interface with colleges and researchers. Recently, my term ended as an executive council member of the NGO (Non-Governmental Organization) Health Committee at the United Nations, but I'm still associated with the committee.

How does the profession differ now from when you first became involved?

I think a significant difference is that almost all of my classmates were either relatives of chiropractors or, like me, had personal experiences with chiropractic that were sufficiently moving to make them want to get this principle to as many individuals as possible.

Some were raised with chiropractic and for them it was just the way you lived life. Others, like me, had a positive chiropractic experience and a desire to bring this to more people.

It's hard not to make a value judgment because I think the impact has been significant and it isn't really anyone's fault, but as prerequisites became more burdensome, the opportunity for potential second career chiropractors diminished significantly.

A lot of people had other careers and because of their chiropractic experience they chose to change. In those days, when there weren't specific science pre-requisites and so forth, it was a relatively easy thing to do. Some people at school with me were in their 60s.

Today, we're getting more individuals who are, for lack of a better term, career shoppers. They're in college or have completed their undergraduate studies and are looking for a career. They may have never been chiropractic patients before. In some schools, a significant majority of incoming students have never had chiropractic as a lifestyle and that has changed the character significantly. There isn't that instant culture, that instant familial relationship we had.

How do chiropractic and performance relate?

Oh, very closely! Chiropractic began, of course, primarily as an alternative means of addressing health problems. Harvey Lillard sought chiropractic care because of his deafness. The second chiropractic patient had a heart condition. Today, most people who seek chiropractic care have some sort of back and neck problem. What many patients and chiropractors have observed over time is that when subluxations are corrected and when people adopt healthier lifestyles, their performance is enhanced.

A limited number of studies have actually looked at athletic performance. There have been numerous anecdotal reports and case studies of individual patients who, as a result of chiropractic care, experienced changes that improved their quality of life. I think we are seeing more emphasis on not just preventing disease but on enhancing function and enhancing performance and thereby improving quality of life. To me, that's really the future of chiropractic. Not the episodic treatment of specific medical issues. We are beyond that.

> *What many patients and chiropractors have observed over time is that when subluxations are corrected and when people adopt healthier lifestyles, their performance is enhanced.*

How does chiropractic relate to a person realizing his or her fullest human potential?

To realize your greatest potential as a human being, you have to have the tool to do that. The tool, of course, is your body. The thing your body uses to process the human experience, the incoming information, and how you react to it, is the nervous system.

As simplistic as it may be, that is the answer. In order to maximize the scope of the human experience, you need a nervous system that's functioning without interference. Therein lies a common problem today in that many people are saying, "Well my problem is stress and I need to eliminate and minimize the amount of stress in my life."

A number of years ago, Hans Selye — who conceived the idea of stress as it related to biological systems — spoke at Palmer. As a faculty member, I had an opportunity to talk with him a bit afterwards. He shared with us a very significant insight, which is in his books: "You do not want to eliminate stress because only a dead person does not make demands on their body." He shared with us that there are two types of stress. One is *eustress*, which is the positive stuff that expands our scope of adaptability and allows us the full range of the human experience.

> *What we as human beings can do that, to our knowledge, other animals cannot, is transmute negative stress or distress into a positive growing experience, by changing our perspective, by changing our attitude, and thereby changing how we respond to it.*

The negative stuff, which he referred to as *distress,* throws us into fight or flight and has deleterious effects on the body, leads to compromised immune function, to cardiovascular disease, to making poor choices regarding food and drink, and substance abuse.

What we as human beings can do that, to our knowledge, other animals cannot, is transmute negative stress or distress into a positive growing experience, by changing our perspective, by changing our attitude, and thereby changing how we respond to it. The idea is not to **eliminate** stress. The idea is to change it to a positive experience that allows you to expand your scope of adaptability. In order to do that, your nervous system needs to be working with no interference. I don't know of any other technology that allows for this except chiropractic.

How does chiropractic offer people an opportunity to realize an enhanced quality of life?

Again, it's all really corollary to the same issue. Essentially, quality of life deals with being able to realize your goals, your dreams, and what you seek out of life. In order to do that, you have to have a clear perception of the world. You need to clearly define your core values and correct any incongruities that exist between your core values and your actions. Finally, you need a body, a mind, and a nervous system capable of realizing the full scope of what you seek and in so doing, your quality of life will be enhanced. What is quality of life about? It's about being able to experience the things you wish to experience in this life without compromise.

What do you feel has happened to the chiropractic profession that may have limited it from being seen by the world in its true nature?

The biggest problem chiropractic has faced is trying to place the square peg in the round hole of third-party pay. It's when chiropractic was included in most insurance programs that the problems began to emerge. In the early days, reimbursement could be received for just about any condition you wanted to put down, although you **did** have to put down a condition.

With time and cost savings becoming a focus of third-party payers, the range of conditions for which they'd reimburse narrowed and finally we have the situation today where they will only reimburse for a narrow sliver of CPT codes related to musculoskeletal pain syndromes.

In order for individuals to obtain reimbursement for chiropractic care, they have to present with a qualifying condition. If your chief complaint is that you aren't able to live life to its fullest, you're not going to get insurance reimbursement whereas if you state that your back or neck hurts, you can. I think that has been responsible more than anything else for limiting full implementation of what chiropractic could be, at least in this country.

Chiropractic has become tagged as a pain relief specialty. In your opinion what more does it have to offer people?

The scope of chiropractic is as broad as the scope of influence of the nervous system, which is the totality of the human experience. I think that pretty well gets it. Pain is certainly a component of quality of life or lack thereof and there is certainly nothing wrong with helping people who are in pain.

There are many individuals who are not in pain, and my concern is that if chiropractic is typecast as a pain-relief specialty and the only way you can get to a chiropractor is if you have a qualifying condition, its potential will never be realized and therefore the potential of humanity will never be realized.

We must make a fierce declaration of independence and purpose, we have to define what we are about, and we have to communicate that. Is it a tall order? Yes, but entirely doable.

When I was in college in the '60s and chiropractic college in the early '70s, many students had spouses who were nurses. In those days, who would have thought that a nurse would be anything other than an assistant to a physician? If you had suggested that registered nurses would one day be able to practice independently, make diagnoses, and prescribe drugs solely on their authority as nurses, people would have said you were absolutely nuts. Yet today, we have nurse practitioners.

It's entirely possible for a profession to reframe itself. It's entirely possible for a profession to have multiple options for people who want to pursue different things. In my work with the U.N., quite frequently I would be asked, "How do you differ from other chiropractors?" and "What is it that chiropractors do?" I told them that some chiropractors choose to specialize in the treatment of musculoskeletal pain while other chiropractors focus on wellness and quality of life. No one is confused by that. If doctors choose to limit their practice to children, to pregnant women, or to people with back pain, that's their privilege. But please, don't limit the profession to one narrow specialty.

What is the purpose of the chiropractic adjustment and how does not receiving chiropractic care impact one's life?

If a person has a subluxation, that subluxation is not correctible by itself. In other words, I think many subluxations are transient phenomenon that spontaneously self-correct. When that *doesn't* happen, and you have a subluxation, the body will do what it does with everything else: utilize its resources to work around it the best it can.

When your life becomes about working around a structural and functional aberration, a tremendous amount of energy is expended, dis-regulation is likely to ensue, and health is going to be compromised.

Do I think nutrition is important? Certainly. Do I think exercise is important? Certainly. Think about this. If a person is subluxated and starts exercising, that exercise is processed through a nervous system designed to work through an aberration. There's training in the memory of the brain and spinal cord, adaptive patterns rather than the patterns that would be manifest without the subluxation. They're setting themselves up for some long-term problems.

What is your favorite quote and how has it impacted your life?

One of my favorite quotes comes from Victor Hugo, who said, "There's nothing more powerful than an idea whose time has come." I adapt that a little bit when I say it because I don't completely agree with it. One thing that's far more powerful than any idea itself is a single individual who has the vision, the passion, and the commitment to make that idea a reality.

How is chiropractic unique and what does it offer that other health professions do not?

The perspective of most health professions is that there is an ever-growing array of diseases out there, as more and more elements of the human condition become medicalized. To them, life is about avoiding these unpleasant conditions that can compromise quality of life and ultimately lead to death. The focus of most health providers is to treat disease, avoid disease, or defer death.

In sharp contrast to that, chiropractic is saying that you needn't be sick to benefit from chiropractic care, you don't have to have an identifiable medical condition to benefit from chiropractic care, and you don't even have to seek to prevent a specific disease or condition to benefit from chiropractic care. All you must have is a desire to express your life to its fullest potential and if you have that desire, the chiropractor can assist you by identifying and correcting areas of interference.

In sharp contrast... chiropractic is saying that you needn't be sick to benefit from chiropractic care, you don't have to have an identifiable medical condition to benefit from chiropractic care, and you don't even have to seek to prevent a specific disease or condition to benefit from chiropractic care.

What do you sense was the intention behind the creation of chiropractic?

It's somewhat difficult to say because D.D. Palmer was a very complex man. He was a magnetic healer before he developed and discovered the concepts of chiropractic. He was an individual who studied the metaphysical realm and spiritualism. It is really difficult to decide whether what he brought forth to the public, and the way he explained chiropractic to the public, was really all he saw or if he merely selectively spun it so it could be consumed by the masses.

Clearly, it was promoted as an alternative treatment for disease. In other words, the idea back then was if you have a disease, rather than go to a medical doctor who is going to do dangerous, possibly deadly, and ineffective things to you, "Come to me, the chiropractor, because I correct the causes of disease."

It began as that, but I can't help but wonder — given his background — whether D.D. didn't see a whole lot more but just didn't feel it was ready for public consumption at the time.

Who are some of your mentors and what impact have they had on your life?

It's difficult to answer that because I am always afraid I'll leave someone out. Obviously, the most significant inspiration, even though I never had the opportunity to meet him, was B.J. Palmer. The thing that impressed me about B.J. was that he was truly a Renaissance man. He is looked upon as being a great philosopher and a great communicator. Few people realize the depth of the individual. He had many diverse interests. He studied religions, eastern philosophies, anatomy, and physiology. He looked at body energy systems. And he was highly committed to developing technology to assess vertebral subluxation and improved methods of correcting it.

B.J. was a true visionary who saw the multi-dimensional aspects of his task, even such things as developing a broadcasting business or opening a printing facility. Whatever it took to get chiropractic to the masses, he did it.

To that end he developed the B.J. Palmer Chiropractic Clinic. He developed instruments such as the Neurocalometer, the Neurocaligraph, the electroencephaloneuromentimograph, three dimensional X-ray analysis protocols, and so forth, all in an effort to get a handle on this thing we call the subluxation, to objectively demonstrate it, and to find better ways to correct it.

He wasn't just a great philosopher, or an articulate orator or an effective salesman. B.J. was a true visionary who saw the multi-dimensional aspects of his task, even such things as developing a broadcasting business or opening a printing facility. Whatever it took to get chiropractic to the masses, he did it.

When he saw opportunities to broaden the application of chiropractic principles, he grabbed it. He purchased Clearview Sanitarium and made it a part of the B.J. Palmer Chiropractic Clinic to call attention to what could be done for individuals with psycho-emotional disorders, psychopathologies, and to provide a training facility for students.

So B.J., of course, is one of the most inspiring. Of people I actually knew, one of the greatest was Fred Barge. Fred was certainly a Renaissance man in his own right in that he wrote books and had a clinic that collected a lot of information concerning the physiology of the body. Many people don't realize that he actually had a clinical laboratory in his office so that he could see what kind of biochemical changes occurred as a result of his care.

He developed chiropractic techniques and equipment. He was president of the International Chiropractors Association and very savvy politically. He was involved in local political issues as well. He was involved in chiropractic education. He spent a tremendous amount of time both at Palmer and Life Chiropractic Colleges lecturing, teaching, and working with key administrators to ensure that chiropractic's true message was perpetuated through the schools. Dr. Barge was certainly an inspiration and my initial contact with him was as a student so I literally knew him throughout my career as a chiropractor and right until he died. He's probably the greatest mentor I had.

Then there are those who are on the cusp and by on the cusp I don't mean by any means lesser, but I'd say that I consider them more of colleague/mentors. These are people such as Guy Riekeman, Patrick Gentempo, and individuals I've had the opportunity to interact and work with. I feel that working with people is more powerful than being alone.

What are some things, if any, you have had to give up in order to devote your life to chiropractic?

I don't really have much of a personal life outside of chiropractic. As I said, most of my friends are chiropractors and most of my non-friends are chiropractors. On the other hand, I have had so many rich opportunities presented to me. Life is always an exchange and it's not so much what you give up as what decisions you make to maximize your effectiveness and to bring you the most pleasure and gratification on a spiritual level, too. Once in a while I think that perhaps I should have had some children; perhaps I should have had a long-term romantic relationship or something like that. Again, I really don't see myself as having given much up because of so much that has been gained.

What turns you on creatively, spiritually, or emotionally?

Probably more than anything else, seeing people "get it" in terms of understanding what chiropractic can do and seeing the passion ignited in them so they can bring it to others.

Where do you see the profession 10 years from now?

We have numerous options, ranging from a glorious future to oblivion and everything in between. Here in the United States we have a health care crisis. It has been written about extensively. It's the focus of the new administration just as it was the focus of the election. We have a so-called health care system that is ready to collapse. The United States spends more money on health care than any other developed nation yet we are very low in the rankings for overall health quality. What in the world is going on?

> **We have some really inspiring scientific evidence showing that individuals who are under long-term chiropractic care utilize fewer medical resources.**

There is a disconnect because the system is based on the wrong premise. It's based on the premise of allowing people to deteriorate until they have a crisis and then "golly gee," we have all these expensive high-tech solutions to get them out of a crisis so they can eek out an existence for a little while rather than die.

What we need is a complete change. We need to shift our focus from dependence on the health care system to individual responsibility. We need a shift from diagnosing, treating, and even preventing disease to empowering individuals to make better life decisions so they can achieve their life potential.

As chiropractors, we have the ability to lead that health care revolution. We have some really inspiring scientific evidence showing that individuals who are under long-term chiropractic care utilize fewer medical resources.

For example, one study found that people over 65 who had received so-called "maintenance" care for five years or more had 50 percent fewer medical provider visits and spent less than a third of the amount of money on medical care than the general population. That is spectacular!

We have evidence that individuals who were in a managed care plan and were permitted to choose a chiropractor as their primary care provider had as much as an 85 percent reduction in prescription drug use.

As I see it, not only can we improve the quality of life of individuals but we can have a major impact, indeed, an impact large enough to significantly mitigate — if not solve — the problem of the failing health care system that's bankrupting our country.

The other possible futures for chiropractic are less desirable. One is to become what some chiropractors think we already are: a narrow medical subspecialty treating primarily non-surgical spinal pain syndromes. Some see that as the desirable niche for the chiropractor. The problem with that, of course, is that the moment you demand that a person have a musculoskeletal condition — one that's on the list to qualify for access to chiropractic care — you have cut off the ability of the majority of humanity to experience its benefits. That's the problem I see.

If a doctor chooses to so specialize, I have no trouble with that. But if the profession unwisely allows itself to be boxed into that niche, I don't see much of a future at all. In fact, I see physical therapy taking over that niche and leaving very little for the chiropractor.

What profession other than your own would you like to have attempted?

I always knew I wanted to be some kind of doctor and I looked at such things as naturopathy. I found that naturopaths were only licensed in a handful of states and when I see the direction that naturopathy is taking today — seeking the ability to prescribe drugs — I'm glad I didn't go that way.

Similarly, I looked at osteopathy or, as it likes to call itself these days, osteopathic medicine. Today, the modern osteopath is virtually indistinguishable from the M.D. Only a tiny handful still accept the tenets and engage in the practices of traditional osteopathy, so I'm kind of glad that I didn't do that.

I was very interested in body-mind stuff. I studied psychology and decided that I'm just not cut out to be a couch jockey. I just didn't see myself doing that. After looking at all of these things, I simply reached the conclusion that there was nothing one human being could do for another that was as safe, that could be delivered as quickly and efficiently, and have as profound an effect on improving a person's quality of life as a chiropractic adjustment.

Not that other things don't have value. It's just that I don't know what else you can do that does that much good in that little time, with that little risk, and for that little money.

Are there any other comments you have about the wonders of chiropractic that you would like to share?

I don't think I can add anything to what I've already said. Someone once said, "Isn't the magnificence of life enough?" I don't know if I can improve on that.

Years from now when people look at your tombstone, what would you want them to read?

This may sound strange but in reality it doesn't matter because my legacy is whatever lives on. It really has little to do with me and it really doesn't matter if they even know who I was if, as a result of my being here, the world is a better place.

↛

Christopher Kent, D.C., FCCI, JD, is the co-founder of the Chiropractic Leadership Alliance. Following graduation from Palmer College, Dr. Kent joined the Palmer faculty, was elected president of the faculty senate, and worked as a principal investigator in the research department.

He moved to Florida to practice full-time, where he qualified as a specialist in chiropractic diagnostic imaging, was named a Fellow of the College of Chiropractic Imaging, and completed visiting fellowship programs in magnetic resonance imaging.

In 1990, he returned to New Jersey to continue research on surface EMG that he had begun several years earlier with colleague and friend, Dr. Patrick Gentempo.

The following year, Dr. Kent received the International Chiropractors Association "Chiropractic Researcher of the Year" award and was again honored by the ICA in 1998 when the organization named him "Chiropractor of the Year."

Elected chair of the United Nations Non-Governmental Organization (NGO) Health Committee in 2001, he was the first chiropractor to hold that office. Dr. Kent was the recipient of the first Lifetime Achievement Award bestowed by Life University.

Larry Markson

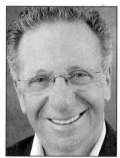

Where are you from originally and what was your childhood like?

I had a typical childhood growing up in Brooklyn, New York. I have a twin brother and we grew up in a chiropractic family starting at age 7. I suffered from bronchial asthma and eczema on my hands that was so bad I had to wear white gloves to school. So my childhood was all about getting well and, thanks to chiropractic, I did. This is what inspired me to become a chiropractor.

Where do you currently reside and how are you spending your time these days?

I live in Boca Raton, Florida and split my time between working with wonderful people in the chiropractic profession, and, of course, playing a lot of golf. For the past two years, my professional focus has been aimed at creating the vision and reality of The Markson Connection. The Vision Statement of the "Connection" clearly explains what it is: "To gather and inspire a tribe of select chiropractors, empowering them to make life-changing decisions that create lives of significance — abundant and overflowing with intention, passion, happiness, and success."

Then, there's my favorite — The Cabin Experience — a personal breaking-free retreat in the middle of a beautiful lake, surrounded by the majestic mountains of Montana. The Cabin Experience is a process by which people can discover who they are and how to unlock themselves from what's holding them back. More than 200 people (only 25 at a time) have experienced it so far and the results are incredible. You can learn more at about it at www.thecabinexperience.com.

How does the profession differ now from when you first became involved?

I became a doctor of chiropractic 48 years ago and, sadly, I think that despite all our advances and technological breakthroughs we have missed the mark in the last dozen years. To me, it seems like chiropractors were more committed and more service oriented in the old days, regardless of the schools they graduated from. Over time, I have witnessed the gradual but important shift in our profession from vitalism to mechanism and from fee-for-service to that of insurance dependence. I have also watched more and more of our colleges adopt a curriculum that has little to do with the chiropractic I know and understand. Where are our principles, the ones that make us a separate and distinct healing art? Why are they no longer taught? Why is the profession moving toward "being accepted" and capitulating to the medical model of health care vs. building a separate heath care model based on our principles?

Many of today's practitioners can't even define chiropractic and their patients never hear the word "subluxation." Patients are dismissed from active care when the pain goes away, when the attorney says so, or when the insurance company no longer reimburses. Some practitioners cannot even intelligently speak about the values of regular chiropractic adjustments as it pertains to the overall health of the human body.

There is a mechanistic and short-sighted view permeating chiropractic right now and I think the profession is struggling because of it. More and more chiropractors are in practice — around 70,000 or so I think — but in my opinion, most of them don't end up earning what I consider to be a professional living from delivering chiropractic as a natural, holistic healing art. Sad to say, but that's what my experience indicates.

As a profession, what do you sense we ought to do to get back on track?

Merge into one powerful national chiropractic organization and do it NOW! The old way hasn't worked and never will. Currently, our three national organizations probably have less than 10,000-12,000 paid members collectively, which means there are still about 55,000 who choose not to be part of any national organization. Why? Because we have been fighting the same fight for the past 25 years and we are getting nowhere.

Practitioners ask, "What are you doing with our money and why are we still where we are after all this time?" Instead, we should be asking, "Where are the regulations, rules, postulates, and positions that define who we are?" How do we get the world to see who we really are? Why don't we fight our battles within one organization and not fight ourselves like we have been doing since the beginning of time? All great questions, I am sure the reader will agree.

The whole profession is looking for recognition, wanting to be more like the medical doctors, to be more insurance dependent, to bill by CPT codes, and to be in hospitals. We want to be known as "doctor" so we can manipulate and treat which, to me, is medicine through the guise of chiropractic.

I don't believe that's what chiropractic is all about and I think the only chance we have to survive is to remain a separate and distinct healing art. Of course, my critics would say that's far too philosophical an approach; that I should get real and keep up with the times. They ask why we can't say manipulation instead of adjustment, why treatment is considered to be a medical word, ignoring the principles that created our profession in the first place.

We are doctors who work with the nervous system and abide by the understanding that the body is a self-healing, self-regulating organism, capable of healing itself from the inside out.

I think chiropractic works on a principle and that principle is natural healing — from the inside out. Chiropractors are not bone doctors or back doctors or neck doctors. We are doctors who work with the nervous system and abide by the understanding that the body is a self-healing, self-regulating organism, capable of healing itself from the inside out.

The body does heal itself which indicates some sort of intelligence within. If we give up the intelligence or spiritual portion of chiropractic, we relegate ourselves to mechanistic manipulating. That's really no different than the MD saying you need to take a pill to get rid of pain — outside in!

I am not denying the place that medicine has in our society — I am saying we, as a profession, are NOT medical doctors. So why then do we attempt to do what they do?

If you're manipulating a spine and not adjusting it and giving credence to the nervous system or some omnipotent force behind it, then you're acting the same way medical doctors do.

Chiropractic is not an acute care healing art and those who practice acute care will only be, in my opinion, in serious jeopardy in the future. The only escape is to practice chiropractic in a model wherein pain relief is only the first part — followed by corrective care and finally the wellness component.

How do you feel chiropractic and performance relate?

I feel the same about chiropractic and performance as I do about chiropractic and general health, emotional stability, internal adaptation, and the general benefits of chiropractic care. If the nervous system is working to the point where the body can adapt to its environment naturally and with effortless ease, then of course performance has to be enhanced. That's why professional athletes utilize the services of chiropractors — and that's why my family and I get adjusted regularly.

How does chiropractic relate to a person realizing his or her fullest human potential?

Now we're talking about philosophy. The extent of human potential is unknown. Years ago, you'd go to the funeral of a 65-year-old man and say he led a long, healthy, and wonderful life, but his time had come. Today, if you went to a funeral for a guy who was only 65 you'd say how sad it is that he passed so young.

Nothing has changed except that human potential is greater today. With a better functioning nervous system, better nutrition, water, and exercise, there's no question we can live into our 90s. Chiropractic care assists in helping all of us reach maximum performance.

How does chiropractic offer people an opportunity to realize an enhanced quality of life?

Quality of life has to do with quality of health. I don't know anyone who is suffering from some sort of malady or breakdown of the body who can be considered healthy. If they're not healthy, they're not happy, and they're not prosperous. When you're healthy, you think better, sleep better, eat better, digest better, and attract into your life more opportunities for higher and greater potential.

What do you feel has happened to the chiropractic profession that may have limited it from being seen by the world in its true nature?

The world doesn't see us in our true nature because we display too many versions of practice and beliefs. Some of my golfing buddies take a pill every day before they play. In fact, they take three Advil or Motrin, put on heat packs and back braces — all before their golf game! When asked why, they say their doctors told them that it would help. Pop a pill and feel better is the model.

Chiropractors advertise on billboards and park benches, they seduce patients by free exams and adjustments, and alter their fees for different patients. So what should we expect in the way of reputation?

Back when I was in practice — and in my son's practice today — more than 50 percent of the patients we attract come to us for health care that has nothing to do with musculoskeletal conditions. Because that is what we promoted, what we taught, and what we believed.

The world today sees us in a very limited way, not as equal to other healing arts. That's sad, but we created it and we earned our own sordid reputation. I'm not blaming the world. I'm blaming us because we don't send out a consistent message — one that tells the true chiropractic story as it should be told.

Chiropractic has become tagged as a pain relief specialty. In your opinion what more does it have to offer people?

It is not a pain relief specialty — that's incorrect labeling. If you want

If the nervous system is working to the point where the body can adapt to its environment naturally and with effortless ease, then of course performance has to be enhanced.

to be out of pain, you can inject drugs strong enough to stop all your pain. Just stick that needle right between your eyes and pull the plunger — it'll knock out your pain and knock you out too. But you won't be healthy — you'll just be out of pain.

Chiropractic isn't about pain; it is about health. Pain is a symptom yelling and screaming, "Ouch, there's something wrong in my body." Chiropractic's job is to find, locate, and remove the cause of that alarm and let the body restore itself from its inability to adapt to its environment.

My belief is that we should devote our time to eliminating all subluxations that interfere with nerve function, so the body can heal itself and get well again. Then I believe the average patient requires follow-up care to stay strong and stay healthy. This is a wellness concept and not just a pain concept. If you stay true to that principle, you'll lose some of the patients you have now, but you would gather a new tribe of people who really want to regain and maintain their health — naturally.

What is the purpose of the chiropractic adjustment and how does not receiving chiropractic care impact one's life?

Chiropractic adjustments are designed to put spinal vertebrae into motion and move them back toward their normal juxtaposition with the vertebrae above and below, while freeing the pressure on the nerves passing through those bony segments.

Not receiving chiropractic care means that the patient will not have the ability to remain free from nerve interference, the end result of which is a lowering of the body's resistance to disease.

This weekend I am babysitting for my grandchildren. One is 4 years old and the other is 6 and they get adjusted regularly. The objective here is to make them as healthy as they can be, to prevent future disease, and to eliminate the micro-trauma they experience everyday.

> **The intention was to create a natural and holistic healing art that recognizes the innate resources of the body to heal itself.**

Chiropractic is a natural healing art that is designed to increase someone's health potential and quality of life by keeping the nervous system functioning at peak performance.

What is your favorite quote and how has it impacted your life?

I'm a big one for sayings and quotes. My favorite of all time has to be, "For every action there is an equal and opposite reaction." That's a Law of Physics and it means the same thing as "What goes around, comes around." What you impress on the inside, you express on the outside. What you put out, you get back — physically, mentally, emotionally, spiritually, and financially.

I like this one, because it places responsibility on me to create the causes of the things I intend to create.

What do you sense was the intention behind the creation of chiropractic?

The intention was to create a natural and holistic healing art that recognizes the innate resources of the body to heal itself. I'm not sure, of course, that D.D. Palmer was aware of any "universal intent" when he gave Harvey Lillard the first chiropractic adjustment. Yet, I do believe that nothing happens without a good reason and there are no mistakes in the Universe. In 1895, that first adjustment was ordained, it was supposed to happen. Chiropractic had to be born for a reason. At least, I have faith in that belief.

Who are some of your mentors and what impact have they had on your life?

I've had many mentors and feel that I have truly been blessed to have had them in my life. I've been adjusted by chiropractic greats like Clarence Gonstead, Arlan Fuhr of the Activator Technique, George Goodheart, Major Dejarnette, and a whole host of chiropractic pioneers.

I have spent time with Jim Parker, Sid Williams, Guy Riekeman, Gerry Clum, Patrick Gentempo, Maurice Pisciottano, countless great management consultants, superstar celebrity speakers, and authors. I have had the pleasure of working with chiropractic college presidents, political gurus past and present, and have come to know and work with most of the leaders of our profession.

But, I guess I consider Dr. James W. Parker to be the most influential person in my personal and professional transformation. He mentored me, coached me, encouraged me, and taught me the Laws of Success. He also told me to hang around with people who were smarter than me in all aspects of life (that's why I am so busy all the time). He taught me to think big, change quickly, be decisive, confront fears, learn something new every day, and to stand up one more time than I was knocked down.

What are some things, if any, you have had to give up in order to devote your life to chiropractic?

I have given up a lot of personal freedom — weddings, confirmations, Bar Mitzvahs, anniversary parties, and family functions — because I lived on the road 25 to 26 weekends a year for many years, working with, learning from, and teaching chiropractors at seminars. I missed a lot of events, yet my family stood behind my concepts and desire to learn and grow.

What turns you on creatively, spiritually, or emotionally?

I'm always turned on creatively, by being able to help others and by positively influencing the chiropractors I have the honor of working with.

Years ago when I was failing personally and professionally as well, I was ready to pack it all in. Then, I changed my mind and learned that it was my attitude that would eventually create the success I was seeking. So, I decided that from that day on I would always be turned on, regardless of life's circumstances.

I learned that successful people had a spiritual connection, were emotionally stable, and didn't bring their past history into their present or their future. They didn't let their history and the past negatives of their lives become their destiny.

I made a decision that from then on I would be spiritually enlightened, emotionally stable, and creatively enhanced throughout my whole life. Right now, at 69 years of age, I am starting a new business. I'm studying, reading, meeting with business coaches, spiritual coaches, and I am, once again, turned on.

Where do you see the profession 10 years from now?

Ten years from now, we'll be okay. It's the next three to five years I am concerned about. I think we're in for some turbulent times. There's going to be a weeding out of the insurance-dependent mechanists and their model of practicing chiropractic. However, I believe that the profession will eventually go on to thrive as a wellness healing art.

The problem right now is that in every other healing art there's a protocol, but every chiropractor practices differently. They have different hours, different fees, different concepts, different techniques, different belief systems, and different staff. Some hold vitalistic views, some hold mechanistic views, and some are "fix and patch." These differences have fractured the profession.

The question should be how to get people to understand chiropractic so when their pain goes away and their insurance goes away, they don't go away. How do we teach them so they stay, pay, refer, and make chiropractic part of their lifestyles so their futures look better?

What profession other than your own would you like to have attempted?

I can't even imagine not being a chiropractor. My experience has been so rewarding and I have loved every second of my career. I would absolutely do it all over again.

Are there any other comments you'd like to share about the wonders of chiropractic?

I have worked with thousands of doctors in the past and the vast majority of them are unique and wonderful. They have created fantastic chiropractic practices, ones that are ethical, honest, and principled. They have great family lives; great relationships with their spouses, their children, and their entire families live a chiropractic lifestyle.

They are tall, small, fat, and thin. There are so-called straights and there are mixers. They are instrument adjusters, hand adjusters, and they believe in chiropractic principles and philosophy. The people I speak of are in total harmony with what's right in the world and they're all miracles to behold.

The true wonder of chiropractic is that there are so many wonderful chiropractors. There are so many people I love and have been fortunate enough to work with and call my friends.

Years from now when people look at your tombstone, what would you want them to read?

He truly cared and he made a difference.

Larry Markson, D.C., personal empowerment, practice success and prosperity coach to more than 25,000 professional offices for the past 28 years, has devoted his professional life to helping doctors and their key assistants transform their thoughts, actions, and feelings until they are able to experience the fulfillment of their life's goals.

He believes that your business, practice and/or your personal life are waiting for a leader (YOU) to show up and that, "Who you are 'inside-the-skin' determines how well what you do works."

Now, in his fifth decade of sharing the secrets of success with audiences all over the world, Dr. Markson has learned that it is successful people who build successful businesses and lives — and that success comes FROM you, not TO you.

Too often we underestimate the power of a touch, a smile, a kind word, a listening ear, an honest compliment, or the smallest act of caring, all of which have the potential to turn a life around.

Leo Buscaglia

Fabrizio Mancini

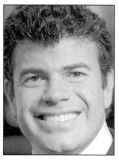

Where are you from originally and what was your childhood like?

I was born in Colombia, South America, in a town on the coast called Barranquilla, which happens to be the same town that the famed singer Shakira is from. My dad's family had one of the largest olive oil, white flour, and pasta companies in my country and in South America. My mom was a school teacher and homemaker and they both came from well known-families with a mentality geared toward healthy self-esteem and making a contribution to society.

I was the fourth of five boys and my childhood was healthy from the perspective that there was a lot of love. My dad always wanted to be a soccer player but, unfortunately, he was the oldest and inherited his father's business at a very young age. He was really never happy at work and retired at 27. I never saw him go to work afterwards.

He made us promise that we would only choose a career we loved and never compromise no matter what. Because of his unhappiness, he began to drink and became an alcoholic. It wasn't until about 10 or 15 years later that I realized he had a drinking problem. He went to a rehab center and for the last 30 years or so of his life he did not have a drink. Unfortunately, he died of lung cancer five years ago due to the fact that, when he was younger, he also smoked from the stress and pressures he felt.

I believe my greatest support has always been my family. My greatest supports from an inspirational standpoint have been my parents, who gave me the values that are my foundation. I have always felt very much loved by my all-encompassing, nurturing, and loving Italian and Colombian family — my brothers, mom and dad, and grandparents — which is the reason that I am the way I am today.

What inspired you to get involved with chiropractic?

I first discovered chiropractic as I was studying pre-med on my way to becoming a neurosurgeon. I had done a rotation in a children's hospital for a year and in surgery and intensive care out of our public hospital for another year. I knew that allopathic medicine was not the answer for the majority of the health problems I was seeing. I felt it was people's thoughts and behaviors that caused most illness. That insight was not reinforced in pre-med or medical school.

I started to recognize that lifestyle behaviors were causing the majority of our health problems. Allopathic medicine was not addressing the problem or the cause of the problem. It was just primarily alleviating the symptoms that were caused by these lifestyle behaviors and attitudes towards health.

What inspired me to get into chiropractic — and continues to inspire and drive me to this day — is my desire to help people understand that unless health is their top priority of values, nothing else will ever fulfill their potential no matter what other values they may have. We're in control of our choices and the choices we make today will determine how healthy we are tomorrow.

Where do you currently reside and how are you spending your time these days?

I live in Irving, Texas and practiced chiropractic here beginning in 1993, having had one of the largest practices in the United States. In 1999, I became president of Parker College of Chiropractic, Parker Seminars, and Parker Share products, which are the three entities I've managed for the last 10 years.

My wife and I have been together more than 20 years. We've been married for 13 years and dated for seven because one of the other things my father instilled in us is that we shouldn't consider getting married until we were 30 years old. He said we'd definitely look at our partner differently and we'd attract someone different at 30 than at 20. He felt we are more stable professionally at that age, so we could really enjoy our family and not feel like our work had a higher priority than our family.

I have two boys, Gianni, 12, and Luciano, 9. I wake up every day at 5:00 a.m. and I'm at the gym by 5:15 a.m. I do various workouts until about 7:30 a.m., get to work by 8:00 a.m., and start meetings at 9:00 a.m. The first six years as president, I would work late because of all of the issues we were facing then. Now that we're very proactive and those earlier challenges have resolved, I can leave around 5:00 p.m.

or so and be home to help my children with their homework or support them in their sports activities, have dinner and just enjoy my time with my wife and kids. As soon as I go through those gates, I shut down my computer and turn off my cell phone. When I'm home, I am a dad, and my role completely changes. I've been fortunate to be able to do that for the past four years very consistently.

How does the profession differ now from when you first became involved?

Right now, the profession is finally beginning to focus in what we agree upon and not what we disagree upon. Some 80-90 percent of all chiropractors agree on the same basic things. We have certain differences of opinion based upon the roots of chiropractic, the history of chiropractic, the education of the schools of chiropractic, and traditionally the viewpoints of our national associations, but we are reaching a point where we recognize we must work as one.

That's the reason Parker Seminars has, for the past three years, had the theme "One Voice for Chiropractic." We all believe we should be delivering one voice and now we have things such as the Foundation for Chiropractic Progress public relations. Over the last three years they have done an amazing job of educating the public about chiropractic and attracting more patients to chiropractors.

Leadership summits are being held twice a year where all our chiropractic leaders discuss issues before they become public. We have become a unified front when it comes to legislative issues and responses to media issues, as well as our efforts to better educate the public and to promote and advance the profession.

When I travel, I see chiropractors all over the world and they don't look any different than in any other country anymore. We need to continue to work as one and continue to support one another regardless of that 10 or 15 percent difference we may feel, because ultimately we must put patients first.

That's one of the things that we at Parker have always supported and promoted. When you put patients first, all of a sudden our small numbers of differences don't become that big of a deal. The most important thing is that people understand and appreciate the value of chiropractic.

How do chiropractic and performance relate?

One of the things that appeals to me about our profession is that it deals with function, which is a very similar word to performance.

The reason why so many high executives, celebrities, and sports people use chiropractic is because they recognize that they do perform better. For the last 20 years, I always get adjusted before I give a speech. I never know in advance what I'm going to say and I believe I perform better when I'm adjusted. I get adjusted once or twice a week because of my travel experience and physical activities.

The unique thing about our profession is that when you are chiropractically evaluated and adjusted, you have the ability to perform at a higher level regardless of where you begin. You may already be performing at a high level but didn't realize you could even go higher. You learn that lesson from working with Olympic athletes. For them, a second or a fraction of a second could mean the difference between a gold or silver medal. It's critical for people to understand that chiropractic automatically allows for a higher level of performance in every area of their lives.

How does chiropractic relate to a person realizing his or her fullest human potential?

If you ask the average person, many would say having headaches every day is normal. Many feel having indigestion after every meal is normal or sleeping three to four hours a day is normal. They think sitting or standing 12 to 13 hours a day is normal. There are a lot of misconceptions regarding what our fullest human potential is.

If you take that to a level of emotional and mental potential, many people think they shouldn't be happy every day and in fact there are people who'll tell you that they don't like people who are happy every day because it makes them feel uncomfortable.

Many people feel relationships are not meant to be long term, where they can really grow with someone. They look at relationships more as a chore or a sentence. It's amazing! I met somebody the other day who told me, "Boy, if my husband ever passes away I'm never getting remarried." I asked her, "What do you mean by that? Isn't being married wonderful?" She said, "Oh, no." Unfortunately, that's how some people feel.

When it comes to the human potential spiritually, many people are very distressed and restless. To me, our physical bodies were meant to be fulfilled, to be productive, to be functioning at a high potential, to be healthy, have healthy immune systems, and healthy nervous systems.

Emotionally, I believe all of us were destined to be happy and find happiness not only in our relationships, but also in our work and everything we do in life. I believe spiritually that we are meant to be at peace and connected with that Universal Intelligence that allows us to be in tune with a higher power, something greater than ourselves.

We need to realize we are just a very small part of something much bigger out there that is amazing. When people recognize the impact chiropractic can have in their lives, they can begin to change their paradigms and realize they were meant to enjoy a greater human potential than they were taught by parents, teachers, and society.

How does chiropractic offer people an opportunity to realize an enhanced quality of life?

The greatest value that chiropractic offers humanity is the ability to have a nervous system that functions better than it did before chiropractic, allowing impulses from the brain to the body and from the body to the brain flow at a very effective pace.

We help the nervous system to function better and that allows the body to heal the way it was designed to. Our body is designed to heal itself, but it can't do that if there is no proper nervous system supporting it.

What do you feel has happened to the chiropractic profession that may have limited it from being seen by the world in its true nature?

As I study the history of chiropractic, I see we have undergone various stages of evolution and the responses to those stages led us to where we are today. In the early days of chiropractic — during the late 1800s to early 1900s — many other professions were starting that were deviations from traditional medicine, such as osteopathy, magnetism, and others. The challenge pioneers like B.J. Palmer faced was to position our profession as unique and counter the attacks that doctors of chiropractic were practicing medicine without a license.

That served a purpose since it accentuated our unique efforts but at the same time it separated us from society's norm. Many people began to look at the chiropractor primarily as a last resort and perhaps even more of a taboo or an esoteric kind of a profession.

In the 1970s, when all of a sudden we started to gain recognition and licensure in every state, we began to appeal to third-party payers to consider reimbursing for chiropractic, which they did. To do that, though, they had to figure out how to fit chiropractic into the insurance system. Third-party reimbursement is always set up primarily on diagnoses based on symptomatic issues, especially related to pain and the relief of symptoms.

Suddenly, a profession that had always been concerned with nerve function and flow rather than symptoms began to play the allopathic game where everything had to be properly diagnosed and properly coded to get reimbursement. In the 1980s, managed care began to change the rules and come up with ways to justify limiting care and decide who had good research to support what they did ... and who didn't.

That's when we began to see some chiropractors return to the traditional premise and say, "Patients have always paid for their services out of pocket because there was value there." But others lost that sense of value because it was just so easy to submit a claim. The patients were coming and the insurance companies were paying. All of a sudden, they saw there was no need to educate patients properly and the profession became like others in healthcare.

> *The reason we are where we are today is because we started with a concept that was way ahead of its time.*

The reason we are where we are today is because we started with a concept and an idea that was way ahead of its time. We are now in a position where our unique approach and our unique philosophy is truly becoming the future of medicine as a whole. Unfortunately, there are other traditional medical disciplines out there trying to claim that they are the innovators and discoverers of this new science, when it has been around since 1895!

Chiropractic has become tagged as a pain relief specialty. In your opinion, what more does it have to offer people?

Chiropractic became more of that primarily because reimbursement by third parties forced us to be more concerned with pain, just as it did with acupuncture in this country. Acupuncture is being embraced, but primarily as a pain reliever.

The story of the first chiropractic patient, Harvey Lillard — a deaf man who regained his hearing through chiropractic — caught my attention because as I studied the nervous system I recognized that when you have a healthy nervous system the body has the ability to heal itself.

Of course, there's always going to be a limitation of matter and healing will depend on how progressed the disease process is, but you always have a better chance of healing when you have a healthy nervous system. I believe that's the message we need to portray out there: if we have a healthy nervous system, the body has a greater ability to heal and function at its highest potential. We have plenty of scientific evidence to support this.

What is the purpose of the chiropractic adjustment and how does not receiving chiropractic care impact one's life?

Primarily, the purpose of receiving the chiropractic adjustment is to restore nerve function and have proper nerve flow. If somebody doesn't receive this gift, they will needlessly continue to suffer the same way they've been suffering. We hear from patients over and over again: "I wish somebody would have told me this was available. It would have saved me all of this pain and suffering, all of this trauma, all of these unnecessary surgeries, and all of these things that have really affected my quality of life."

What is your favorite quote and how has it impacted your life?

I have many, but my favorite is from Albert Einstein: "You cannot solve the problems of today with the same level of thinking that created them." I love that quote because it reminds me that, when something isn't working and I'm being challenged, the first thing I must do is change my level of thinking. That's what created the problem in the first place and I need to begin to think or look at things from a different perspective.

How is chiropractic unique and what does it offer that other health professions do not?

The fact that chiropractic focuses on nerve intervention makes it unique since we have other professions promoting natural healing and better lifestyle behaviors. Chiropractic can promote all of that but if a nervous system is subluxated, is interfered with, and is not allowing the body to function to its highest potential, the person will never be as healthy as he or she was meant to be. I think that is our uniqueness.

What do you sense was the intention behind the creation of chiropractic?

I've read D.D. Palmer's texts and know he was very interested in and passionate about electromagnetic forces. I believe he felt that, through chiropractic, he could actually impact electromagnetic forces — our nerve flow — in a way that was practical, in a way that was very powerful, in a way that was cost-effective, and in a way that was life changing. I think he succeeded. To this day, I haven't found a health care profession that can offer what we offer to patients in such a practical, inexpensive, cost-effective, and powerful way just by delivering the chiropractic adjustment.

Who are some of your mentors and what impact have they had on your life?

I would have to start with my mom and dad because of the way they raised me with so much love and nurturing, with such great values, and to show sensitivity and responsibility toward others.

When I entered chiropractic, Dr. James W. Parker really became my strongest mentor because I saw in him an individual who truly dedicated his life, in every way, to promoting and advancing the profession while helping other chiropractors fulfill their dreams in chiropractic. I also saw he was focused intently on helping patients fulfill their health dreams through chiropractic. He was a dedicated person, yet it cost him four marriages because of the imbalance of dedicating his life to traveling all over the world, speaking everywhere, and being gone much of the time from his family. To his dying day, I know he wished he would have had a little more balance in his life. That has been a great lesson for me and I remind myself of it every single day.

> **I wake up every day thankful to be alive and have the ability to contribute, and thinking about how I can contribute at a high level.**

Through Dr. Parker and Parker Seminars, I met Dr. John Demartini, who amazed me with his passion, his desire to help and inspire so many, his desire to travel the world to share with others this great message of ours, and tell them of the incredible potential they have as individuals if they choose to access it.

Jack Canfield and Mark Victor Hanson were speakers at Parker and I became very well acquainted with them when we did our "Chicken Soup for the Chiropractor's Soul" project together. It was a wonderful experience to work side by side with these gifted individuals.

I was the chiropractor for Dr. Phil McGraw for many years and to this day he is still a mentor because of his desire to impact people and help them deal with very difficult issues.

From an historical perspective, I've always looked at the lives of Mother Teresa, Gandhi, Martin Luther King, Jr., Nelson Mandela, and Muhammad Ali as some of my greatest influences. These people truly were tested by time and persevered through all challenges confronting them because they believed they were here to help advance a cause they believed in. These are the people who truly allow circumstances around them to define them in a positive way. Unfortunately, some of them died tragically but they left a legacy behind that inspired millions of people to support something worth supporting.

What are some things, if any, you have had to give up in order to devote your life to chiropractic?

Chiropractic has given me everything I have in my life. It's given me a tremendous ability to be healthy. It's given me the ability to have a healthy relationship with my spouse, children, and family. The one thing that I *have* had to give up because of the role I'm serving right now is full-time practice, which is something I truly loved. Being with patients every day was wonderful. The fulfillment I get right now by inspiring the lives of thousands of students here, so they can go out and help people through chiropractic, definitely fills that void but I do feel like I gave up something I truly loved. I still adjust quite often but not to the degree while I was in practice full-time. I would say that's the only thing I've had to give up because of my current role. I feel that I've gained everything else because of chiropractic.

What turns you on creatively, spiritually, or emotionally?

There's one thing that does that more than anything and that is to serve. I have this thing (and my mom says I have had it since I was a little boy): I never waste a single day. I wake up every day thankful to be alive and have the ability to contribute, and thinking about how I can contribute at a high level. All of a sudden, I'm asked to do things that allow me to do just that. One doesn't get to be where I am by *choosing* to be in this position. That's one thing I've learned. You get to be where I am now, and wherever I will be in the future, by dedicating your life to service for others and contributing at high levels.

Where do you see the profession 10 years from now?

Right now, we have some of the greatest opportunities that chiropractic has been offered in many years. The Association of Chiropractic Colleges' productive meetings over the last three to five years to try to harmonize chiropractic education across the board are a positive step. The intention is to have schools not look so different from one another just for the sake of trying to preserve some tradition or because of their founders, etc.

This situation is getting much better and will ultimately produce more well-balanced chiropractors who will not look that different from their colleagues who graduated from somewhere else. I think that's critical.

I think it is also critical that the International Chiropractors Association and American Chiropractic Association are working together better than ever and that the Congress of Chiropractic State Associations and the state associations are working better than ever together. They have regular meetings and they really have a great and balanced leadership, which is a wonderful thing.

My greatest satisfaction is seeing people coming into this profession who are of much higher quality, from a health perspective. They're healthier, younger, and more balanced by gender (we now have 42 percent females across the board in chiropractic education).

We have greater diversity in that we see more Hispanic-Americans, African-Americans, Asian-Americans, Indian-Americans, etc. and I think that allows us to fill the gaps in those communities where there aren't enough chiropractors.

Chiropractic is growing by leaps and bounds outside of the U.S. There are more colleges now outside the U.S. than inside, and a lot more will open within the next five years. We are going to see a tremendous growth of more licenses and more colleges. Right now, we have 92 chiropractic associations affiliated with the World Federation of Chiropractic — 92 different countries and more are joining every day.

Another great opportunity is the fact that we are trying to position ourselves now, when a new administration in the U.S. is looking for solutions to our health care crisis. Our profession is positioned to be a great part of that solution if we can secure greater participation within our health care system. Hopefully, our legislators in Washington will see the logic of that and the only challenge we have is fighting a tremendous amount of lobbying from the pharmaceutical companies that don't want to give up their revenue source.

At some point, they're going to have to ask, "Is this worth killing our people?" and "Is this worth maintaining and supporting the continuation of our people suffering every single day?" At that point, I hope their hearts will speak louder than the special interests and they will do the right things for the public. We have shown over and over again the tremendous value chiropractic has if it's utilized more effectively across the board.

What profession other than your own would you like to have attempted?

Initially, my journey was kind of interesting. When I was 17 years old, I had a dream that I was going to become a doctor. I believe my inspiration came from my pediatrician, which was the type of doctor I thought I wanted to become. This is the reason that in pre-med I did a year of rotation at Children's Hospital here in Dallas. I then realized that I love children too much and the hospital was not the right environment for me. I felt perhaps there was another way I could help them. I became very passionate about the nervous system and this is when I started moving more towards neurosurgery. I then did a year of rotation in neurosurgery but I realized that arena was too mechanical — I believe the nervous system is far more powerful than that.

As surgeons, all I felt we were doing was repairing what had already been damaged but not really helping people appreciate and preserve what is already naturally given: a beautiful and healthy nervous system. Those were really the only other considerations that I have had in my life. I've been a chiropractor since 1990 and have never thought about anything other than just being a chiropractor.

Are there any other comments you'd like to share about the wonders of chiropractic?

When people ask where I see chiropractic in the future, I always say that chiropractic in the future will look exactly the same way you are choosing to express chiropractic within yourself and your practice — except multiply it by 75,000.

If all of us choose to practice chiropractic in the way it was destined to be practiced — with the purest of intentions and a sense of hope rather than the sense of despair, with a sense of vitalism rather than the sense of mechanism, with a sense of truly appreciating what is God-given and treasuring the Innate Intelligence within us — then chiropractic will be exactly what everybody wants it to be.

It all depends on what we do every single day of our lives and how we choose to practice. If you want chiropractic to be doom and gloomy, then keep being doom and gloomy yourself. If you want chiropractic to thrive and prosper, then you thrive and prosper and you will inspire others to thrive and prosper until, hopefully, we get to the point where we can all thrive and prosper in this profession.

Years from now when people look at your tombstone, what would you want them to read?

It's so funny because my wife and I have talked about that. When I lived in Rome, I had the opportunity to visit the city of Assisi and got a chance to really understand the life of St. Francis of Assisi. St. Francis has a prayer which has always been the way I want to live my life and the way I hopefully will be remembered. When I first read it, it didn't have as much meaning to me; it was simply something that was nice to read. Eventually, it became kind of a life mission to me. It is:

"Lord, make me an instrument of Thy peace;
Where there is hatred, let me sow love;
Where there is injury, pardon;
Where there is doubt, faith;
Where there is despair, hope;
Where there is darkness, light;
And where there is sadness, joy.

"O Divine Master,
Grant that I may not so much seek
To be consoled, as to console;
To be understood, as to understand;
To be loved as to love.

"For it is in giving that we receive;
It is in pardoning that we are pardoned;
And it is in dying that we are born to eternal life."

I want people to feel that my life was dedicated to all of the things that prayer encompasses. I have it always around me and it's one of the greatest inspirations to me.

Upon graduation from Parker College of Chiropractic in 1993, **Fabrizio Mancini, D.C.,** launched the Mancini Chiropractic Center in Dallas. Just six years later, he was asked to head Parker College, making him the youngest college president ever in the United States.

Dr. Mancini has given testimony to the White House Commission for Complimentary and Alternative Medicine and has served for years on the Texas Governor's Advisory Council on Physical Fitness. He has been inducted in all three fellowships as a Fellow for the International College of Chiropractors, the American College of Chiropractors, and the International Chiropractic Association.

The list of numerous awards he has received includes: Humanitarian Award, Heroes for Humanity Award, Chiropractor of the Year Award, CEO Award, Vision Award, High-Spirited Citizen Award, Rising Star Award, Crystal Apple Educators Award, Extra-Ordinary Speaker Award, Award of Honor, Who's Who, ACA and TCA President's Award, and others. Dr. Mancini has been inducted into the Wellness Revolutionaries Hall of Fame for his contributions in this field.

CJ Mertz

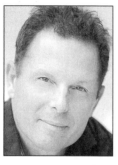

Where are you from originally and what was your childhood like?

I'm originally from northern California, having grown up in San Jose. My childhood was phenomenal! I grew up in a household that really was modest financially but my siblings and I never felt like we missed anything. Anytime I needed some cleats or a tennis racquet, they always seemed to show up. My dad worked many graveyard shifts just to make certain we had the kind of life he wanted to see for us. He was an amazing father and is still largely my role model today. My mom was the glue for our family and we all shared wonderful family ties that exist even now. The close relationship I have today with my brothers and sisters is evidence of how we were raised and how we came together as a family during my childhood.

What inspired you to get involved with chiropractic?

I had a very bad football injury when I was playing in a Pop Warner league when I was 10. I was punting the ball and a player from the other team came in to block the punt and I actually wound up kicking him. He came between my foot and the ball and they took him off in a stretcher, which is an indication of how badly he got hurt. Something jarred in my back and at first I didn't feel any pain, just heat.

I told my coach about it when I got to the sidelines and he put some "icy-hot" on my back, which of course was already hot, so it was now flaming. I went in on the next series of plays on defense, intercepted the ball, and got hit from the front and back. This time I was taken off on a stretcher.

I was in the hospital with my mom on a Saturday and the test results showed two crushed vertebrae and a crushed disc. I couldn't feel much in my legs at this point and I felt no pain other than this outrageous heat sensation.

They told my mom they wanted to do surgery and I would probably get most of the feeling back in my legs although I would probably have a little wobble in my walk. They also said that my spine would deteriorate much more quickly than other people and I would never play sports again.

My mom immediately made two phone calls on this big rotary phone in the room. She called my dad first and then she called her chiropractor. That was the key right there: that my mom somehow had the wisdom — and had been given enough from her chiropractor — that at that hospital, on a Saturday, she knew to call her chiropractor.

He told my mom to get me in the station wagon, take any X-rays and files with us, and get me out of the hospital. Against all the doctors' recommendations, she took me out of there. I distinctly recall being at the chiropractor's office looking at the X-rays from the hospital. He took his own X-rays as well, and we also looked at the MRIs and other files. He told my mom that my condition was as bad as they'd said it was. He told her he wanted to start working with me for 30 days and if he couldn't help me, there was a chiropractor about an hour north who was more specific and better with this than he was. If the other chiropractor couldn't help either, then they'd send me to the middle of the country to the doctor he thought was the finest chiropractor in the world. If all that was to no avail, he'd recommend I go back to the hospital where we started so they could do the surgery.

As a 10-year-old boy, what I really learned was: chiropractic first, chiropractic second, chiropractic third, and at the very last, if nothing else worked, then try surgery.

We started working together and I was a little bit better in 30 days, even better in 60 days, and six months later I was hopping, skipping, and jumping. That was how I started my journey in chiropractic. I will never forget being on the swing and looking at my legs, just so excited that I was fully healed.

I remember saying to my chiropractor, when he walked into the room six months later to give me my adjustment, "Doc, thank you so much for giving me my legs back."

He put his fingers to my chest and told me, "Son, don't ever say that again." My heart sank to my stomach wondering why he said that, after I just paid him a compliment the only way a boy could.

What he said next is the reason I became a chiropractor. He said, "I want you to remember for the rest of your life that I moved the bone but God did the healing." He taught me dearly about subluxation but he did not want me to think he healed me. I remember going home and talking to my mom, saying something like, "Mom, wouldn't it be cool if some day I could do this and help another child?" There was a seed planted right there and then.

Where do you currently reside and how are you spending your time these days?

I spend my time in Austin, Texas, with my beautiful bride Andrea (who is the daughter of Kirby Landis, a legend in chiropractic) and our three angels: Chandler, 10; Cody, 8; and Cailyr, 6. They're my world and that is what I do. They're involved in everything you could imagine — dance, swimming, gymnastics, golf, tennis, and Tae Kwon Do. I'm there cheerleading, mentoring, and loving them. That's what I do when I'm not traveling, teaching seminars, or coaching chiropractors. I'm also very disciplined with my workout regimen and I love to play golf.

How does the profession differ now from when you first became involved?

When you say the profession, the first thing that comes to my mind is the chiropractors themselves because to me the profession is the chiropractors and the patients. When I think about the chiropractors, CAs, and patients, what I notice is sort of what my dear friend Gerard Clum from Life West Chiropractic College said a few years ago, that chiropractic is like a tale of two cities. That's what I see here. I see, on one hand, chiropractors who have just left the philosophical foundation. At least four out of 10 chiropractors don't even have an X-ray machine, so even their sense of the way they go about the work-up and continued evaluation of the patient has changed.

I think the overall desire has changed. When I think back 25 years ago, many chiropractors had a burning desire to have 300 patient visits a week, helping countless men, women, and children. It was common and you could see palpable desire in those chiropractors.

The most successful principled practices I have ever seen are being built right now but I'm also seeing more chiropractors failing in practice than ever before. It's almost like Middle America chiropractic is disappearing. There's a fork in the road where chiropractors either go quickly to mere survival, struggling, or failing altogether, or they go to a place of tremendous prosperity, success, and growth.

That dichotomy is interesting. I think the reason for this split is that 25 years ago you could make a certain number of mistakes and still succeed. There are essentially five core components to the success of a chiropractor. Twenty-five years ago, a chiropractor could be above average in two of those and still succeed very well. Today, chiropractors really need to be above average in at least three or four in order for them to have the same level of success they would have had then. The level and depth of training for the average chiropractor has not improved, but the standard has.

How do chiropractic and performance relate?

I think chiropractic is the study of human performance. Chiropractic is the art, science, and philosophy of human performance because there is no performance of the body without nerve supply and there's no performance without function.

It doesn't matter if we're talking about top athletes, people who are just incredible at their trades, or parents taking care of their children. Certain levels of performance are needed by all of these, and chiropractic offers human beings the opportunity to perform at their best by having the right information traversing the nerve system so that what the mind perceives the body doing, the body can actually fulfill.

How does chiropractic relate to a person realizing his or her fullest human potential?

Human beings have been given a genetic code and that code gives them the amazing ability to be all that God intended them to be. Chiropractic gives people the chance, through the Innate Intelligence that runs and operates their bodies, to reach that highest level of potential.

Perhaps the individual child has Downs Syndrome or we're working with an Olympic athlete in another instance. In either case, chiropractic can bring out the very best that person is capable of, because without the proper ratio and flow of nerve supply and proper intelligence to the cellular level, the body will never have a chance to excel and get to the level of achieving its full genetic and God-given potential.

How does chiropractic offer people an opportunity to realize an enhanced quality of life?

What's so amazing about chiropractic is that what we do is NOT a treatment. Chiropractic offers a lifestyle (an awesome word!) because it offers a paradigm. Chiropractic isn't just something you do but something you believe and think about. You find the lifestyle within its philosophy.

When you think about the quality of someone's life and how chiropractic plays a part in that, you'll see how huge a part it plays, because it offers a wellness lifestyle. Living that lifestyle, people make vacation choices geared towards health and wellness, increase their water intake, move their body more, make healthier food choices, and get adjusted every week.

We now see people doing things within a chiropractic lifestyle to bring them greater strength, balance, excellence, coordination, and memory. In many ways, chiropractic defines quality of life and leads to enhanced quality of life by offering the opportunity of a lifestyle.

What do you feel has happened to the chiropractic profession that may have limited it from being seen by the world in its true nature?

I have to give you a small story for this one. When I was in elementary school — and I remember like it was yesterday — a bus rolled up to school and this big Russian woman came out of it and into our classroom. She looked seven feet tall to us second graders. She came in the class and I don't remember her even saying "hi." I just remember her saying in this loud Russian voice, "If you don't brush, they'll rot!"

Of course, she was talking about teeth and we were taken out of our class onto her little bus where there were all of these little sinks with mirrors on the wall. She gave each of us a little red pill and she said to us, "Brush until it's gone!"

We're brushing like crazy and fighting for our lives with this seven-foot Russian woman and I noticed that even with brushing like crazy the red was still there — but it was from my bleeding gums because of brushing too hard!

The whole thing was absolutely frightening, but I will tell you that after that experience I've continued to brush my teeth twice a day since. What chiropractic is missing is a large Russian woman.

What happened in second grade was part of a grass-roots movement that the dental profession figured out but chiropractic hasn't. We're missing the little red pill: the ability for children starting in elementary school to hear about subluxation, to hear about Innate Intelligence, to understand the significance of posture and how that relates to spinal hygiene.

With that, we would see chiropractors become recognized for who and what we are. Unfortunately, we've never done that and as a result we're still locked in the neck-and-back-pain box. What the public should realize about what we do is that we serve the human being and the way chiropractic has been sold to and accepted by the public up to this point is a lie.

Chiropractic has become tagged as a pain relief specialty. In your opinion what more does it have to offer people?

We spoke about lifestyle a moment ago and that's really where chiropractic is moving: a lifetime strategy, a lifetime sense of confidence, and a lifetime tool and solution for families. Chiropractic needs to be viewed as the lifetime family wellness solution. Not until these three words — lifetime family wellness — become synonymous with chiropractic will we reach our pinnacle. The average chiropractor sees what I refer to as "broken families." Maybe a mom comes in, but no other members of the family do. Or, one child gets adjusted but no one else from the family does. I want to give credit to the many hundreds of chiropractors who do have whole families come in to get adjusted and live the lifestyle. That's what it's all about, lifetime family wellness and that's where it needs to go.

About 97 percent of the people who come to a chiropractor, unfortunately still in this day and age, come for some relief of a condition. Therefore, the relationship between a person and chiropractic starts off conditionally and that's where we need to see the breakthrough.

Chiropractic was never designed to be conditional and was not for the purpose of treating a symptom or a condition. It was designed to be a solution for healing and healing is a process. The body itself is a process and the body is constantly repairing and breaking down. That's as true in the child as it is in the adult.

We go through the developmental processes from infancy to childhood to adolescence to adulthood and through all of these phases the body requires a level of healing that allows for a level of repair and homeostasis. In the chiropractic model, the lifestyle and philosophy of chiropractic enters right into that place where the mom and her needs, the dad and his needs, and the children and their needs are congruent because all of them — although in different phases and different developmental areas of life — have one thing in common: their bodies heal exactly the same.

What is the purpose of the chiropractic adjustment and how does not receiving chiropractic care impact one's life?

The purpose of a chiropractic adjustment is to maintain 100 percent nerve supply within the body and the philosophy of chiropractic reminds us that the power that made the body heals the body. The chiropractor isn't responsible for the healing. The chiropractor is responsible for making sure there is no interruption to the source that's responsible for all of the healing.

That adjustment should be happening on at least a weekly basis because life is the main cause of the subluxation. All too often, people think subluxations are caused by auto accidents, athletic injuries, or some other traumas. Those things do cause vertebral subluxations, but really the planet is affecting us every day through stresses, toxicities, and through traumas (emotional, physical, and otherwise). Life itself is enough of a reason for the creation of the lessening of or interruption to the very nerve system that controls and operates our entire body.

Getting adjusted regularly and allowing the effect of those adjustments to accumulate maximizes function and maximizes the body's ability to adapt to its environment. That's why we often see children who get chiropractic stay well even though the flu bug is going around school. Chiropractic has the ability to assist in their enhanced adaptation to the environment. They're able to adapt better to temperature changes and all the other various things that happen in their lives because of the adjustments.

What is your favorite quote and how has it impacted your life?

Quite frankly, there are so many as I am an excessive reader and studier. I have followed so many great mentors, authors, and teachers over the years. If I were to bring it down to just a couple, the first would be Gandhi's, "Be the change you wish to see in the world." I love that one because it brings all of it back to an inside-out model. If you want to see more love in the world, be more loving yourself. If you want to see more prosperity, then be more prosperous, kinder, more loving, and more patient — whatever it may be for that individual. I also think what Gandhi reminded us when he said, "To eat simply so that others may simply eat," is wonderful.

How is chiropractic unique and what does it offer that other health professions do not?

We have talked about the term *lifestyle* and I will just go back to that. I believe what chiropractic offers that no other health profession offers is a living paradigm. Within that, people can start to make sense of their lives so things are not simply *coincidental* or so separate that they need a pill or a potion for every different thing that goes on whether it's an anti-inflammatory, antibiotic, or pain killer for each separate ailment.

There are so many different thoughts, ideologies, and treatment methods. Yet, chiropractic allows people to actually build faith, confidence, and beliefs about the structure God has created called "themselves." With it, they understand that the body can heal itself. Chiropractic has created a paradigm for people to think about life, family, and health in a way that allows them to make better choices. To me, that's what separates chiropractic from everything else.

What do you sense was the intention behind the creation of chiropractic?

D.D. Palmer stated it as well as or better than anyone I've ever studied or read. He said the purpose of chiropractic is to "unite man the physical with man the spiritual." More than 100 years ago, D.D. used the word *tone*. He said the body was given a gift, and the gift is that God has created within us a certain vibration and that state of vibration is the optimum state of being. He called it tone.

We are all mental, physical, and spiritual beings with a certain vibrational state. When we are at the optimum state of being, we have the greatest joy, greatest human experience, greatest quality of life, and greatest quality of function as a human being. The key is to be able to find and stay in that tone. I truly believe that was the intent.

> **We are all mental, physical, and spiritual beings with a certain vibrational state. When we are at the optimum state of being, we have the greatest joy, greatest human experience, greatest quality of life, and greatest quality of function as a human being.**

Who are some of your mentors and what impact have they had on your life?

First and foremost is our Lord Jesus Christ. He is my number one mentor and through him all things are possible. He has saved and carved my life, while giving it purpose.

I also hold B.J. Palmer as a tremendous mentor. This includes all of his Green Books and all his teachings, which have been absolutely sensational and helped me develop my own confidence and understanding about chiropractic and the world.

I've also taken much high-level training coursework in personal development. Tom Peters, author of "In Search of Excellence" and so many other incredible books, is a leadership mentor. There is, of course, Stephen Covey as well, who wrote "The Seven Habits of Highly Effective People." These two men have been very personally rewarding in my life and have helped shape many of my thoughts and actions.

I also want to thank Dr. Don Harrison, founder of Chiropractic Biophysics, who very early in my career was a fantastic technical mentor inside chiropractic. And I want to include my father, Vincent Mertz, who just really showed me how to be a good man.

What are some things, if any, you had to give up in order to devote your life to chiropractic?

It's the complete opposite for me. To sum up in one word what I have given up would be: laziness. I think it's certainly true for anybody but definitely for me that in order to really excel, I had to be able to give up a strong tendency to just chill, hang out, be lazy, sleep in, not study, or not take something to the next level. Laziness is something that I had to give up. It's certainly been a worthwhile tradeoff, I will tell you that.

What turns you on creatively, spiritually, or emotionally?

Leading others to a change in their core beliefs and in their core habits. Witnessing a chiropractor, patient, friend, or neighbor see himself or herself and the world differently. Changing and improving somebody's beliefs, watching the lights come on inside the person, and seeing the literal change in his or her habits as a result of that — so it's not just a new thought but actually a new response to that belief. I would say that's the most emotionally fulfilling and spiritually fulfilling act.

Where do you see the profession 10 years from now?

I'm one of the few teachers and coaches who travel internationally every year. I travel throughout the United States, Canada, Europe, Australia, and Asia and I see chiropractic growing outside of the United States at an unprecedented rate, which I couldn't have said a decade ago.

I know this will probably surprise you but what I see 10 years from now are on-purpose chiropractors from outside the United States actually thinking about going on a mission here.

I see people from Singapore doing a chiropractic mission in Nashville. I see chiropractors from various places in the world coming in and doing a mission in L.A. or going right into Miami and other places simply turning whole cities on to chiropractic because chiropractors in the United States have lost the sense that there is a mission.

What profession other than your own would you like to have attempted?

I would love to have been the pastor of a large church. That would have been really fulfilling.

Are there any other comments you'd like to share about the wonders of chiropractic?

Chiropractors must always come back to the understanding that chiropractic is perfect and that chiropractic always works. We can never limit the principle of chiropractic nor can we ever limit the human body's ability to literally resurrect itself because of the power that was gifted inside of it.

We see chiropractors today doing incredible things for children who have autism. We see incredible things happening with remissions in people who have multiple sclerosis. When we see cancer being put into remission, eyes regaining sight, and hearing restored, we can never simply reduce chiropractic to our current reality. If I focus only on the back pain, neck pain, and headaches coming into my practice, that's what I'll attract back. It becomes a self-fulfilling prophecy. Chiropractors have to go out of their box and be able to see what is really true. When they do that they're able to truly see the wonders and miracles chiropractic is capable of and was designed to be part of.

Years from now when people look at your tombstone, what would you want them to read?

I would absolutely want them to read: "Here lies CJ Mertz, a loving husband, a loving father, and a loving servant of the Lord." That's what I have manifested in my life. Anything else that would be written there regarding my legacy or anything else in chiropractic probably has more to do with other people figuring that out. I'll leave that to someone else.

ॐ

CJ Mertz, D.C., who by age 28 had built one of the largest subluxation-care family practices, realized that for subluxation to become a household word, chiropractors needed to be leaders of their communities. In 1984, Dr. Mertz (known throughout the profession as "Coach CJ") founded The Waiting List Practice (Team WLP), an organization that trains chiropractors with a systematic approach to running successful, subluxation-centered care practices.

Traveling nearly three million miles, Coach CJ has trained more than 10,000 chiropractors and opened over 3,000 subluxation-based chiropractic practices. He has also produced and developed a world-class infomercial, patient education material, and the first fully-automated, paperless chiropractic office system.

Dr. Mertz was voted "Teacher of the Year" in 1986, "Chiropractor of the Year" in 1995 and "Humanitarian of the Year" in 2001. In 2002, he was named president of the first chiropractic franchise, publicly held Chiropractic USA. In 2003, he was elected the 14th president of the International Chiropractors Association.

Jeanne Ohm

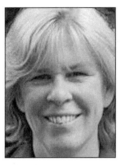

Where are you from originally and what was your childhood like?

I'm from Long Island, New York. My childhood was typical of someone growing up in the '60s and '70s. I came from an upper middle class family. My father was an insurance salesman, so we had health insurance back then, although most families did not. I actually had three major surgeries by the time I was 6 because it was covered. We had the typical medical care and American lifestyle —and then I met my husband Tom's family.

They were completely different, in how they approached health. When his father had a fever he'd put on 10 layers of clothes and go under the covers so he could "sweat it out" and go to work the next day. They never went to the medical doctor, and they did their "minor surgeries" on the kitchen table.

When Tom and I were 19, we were living together with his brothers and we went out hang-gliding. I fractured my spine and took the medical route: drugs, orthopedic brace, exercise — the full gamut. I remember returning to the orthopedic surgeon a year after the accident and telling him, "My back still hurts!" He said to me, "Honey, you're going to have a bad back for the rest of your life." I told myself — and him — that there was no way that would be the case! I walked out (crying) not knowing what I was going to do.

What inspired you to get involved with chiropractic?

Somebody suggested I go to a chiropractor because they heard chiropractors worked with the back. I walked into this chiropractic office, and the chiropractor told me that I would receive no care until I sat with Tom for one of his lectures. His chiropractic assistant at the time was Rose Panico. She was sitting there, enthusiastically talking about chiropractic, and we were wondering what all the passion was for. Our chiropractor got very deep and philosophical in the lecture, explaining that chiropractic dealt with reducing interference in the nervous system so the body can express itself and we as beings could express who we really were. I was thinking, "Just fix the back problem."

Three months later after very regular care, my allergies, asthma, and migraine headaches were gone, and my menstrual cycle was regular. I asked him what he was doing, because nothing else had changed in my life. He said, "Remember what I initially I told you, your body is a self-healing organism that needs interferences removed."

He then asked us what we were doing with our lives. He told Tom to become a chiropractor and he suggested I could be the chiropractic assistant. Sparked by what we were learning and its consistency with our personal philosophies, we started attending numerous chiropractic gatherings. They focused on philosophy and the principle of chiropractic.

During one of those meetings, somebody read a B.J. Palmer quote that really resonated with our personal beliefs. It was: "In our hasty thinking to secure an education, we are prone to say I am a body with a soul. Rather we should say and think, I am that innate intelligence with a body in which to express myself." Tom and I looked at each other and said that if that's really what the foundation of this profession is about, we're in!

We considered Life College, Sherman College of Straight Chiropractic, and ADIO. We went to ADIO because it was close to New York. The name later changed to Pennsylvania College. It was pretty crazy there, wrought with political struggles, but as for the education for chiropractic, we were palpating spines on the second day of class and were adjusting in the second quarter.

Where do you currently reside and how are you spending your time these days?

We live outside Philadelphia and have six children, all whom were born at home. Our youngest is 16, so we are on the other end of raising kids. We are now entering the stage of daughters-in-law and grandchildren. We have a home office; it was our way to stay as close as possible as family while the kids were young. To this day, a big part of our time is spent together as family. We've been in practice for over 25 years, and have had a family practice right from the start.

Our oldest son, Justin became a chiropractor as well, and currently he and Tom see most of the patients. I'm not in the office except for some specific children's and pregnancy cases where people just insist that I see them.

Otherwise, every weekday I work with the International Chiropractic Pediatric Association (ICPA), which was founded by Dr. Larry Webster about 25 years ago. It isn't affiliated with any political organization. It's non-profit and we do research, training, and public education. We're currently doing some phenomenal children's research projects. We hold about 180 classes all over the world every year. We offer the largest certification and Diplomate program in pediatrics and maternal wellness.

The ICPA has three websites. One for doctors, one for public education, and one for our full-color print magazine, *Pathways to Family Wellness*. *Pathways* is my newest little baby — it recently had its five-year anniversary. It's now on the racks at Barnes & Noble and Borders, making it the first chiropractic family wellness magazine to reach major newsstands. We are pretty psyched about that.

As executive director of the ICPA, I oversee all of the above departments. In addition, on weekends I travel internationally teaching chiropractors how to adjust pregnant mothers and infants. That covers about seven days a week most of the year. I do take the summer weekends off to be home with the family.

How does the profession differ now from when you first became involved?

When I first became involved, it was grounded in philosophy and a confirmation of a bigger vision. We understood the concept of vitalism through chiropractic philosophy well before the word vitalism became "popular."

After graduating, I remember going to a meeting where everyone was talking about how insurance coverage was coming down the pike. People were saying how wonderful that would be, and one old chiropractor got up and said that this was the worst thing that could ever happen to us. The place got dead quiet and people couldn't understand why he said that. In retrospect, I believe he was right. We stepped into that whole mechanistic paradigm and caused confusion in consumers' minds leading them to interpret us as just another treatment for conditions, natural though it may be.

On a physical level, chiropractic restores communication between brain and body, allowing the body to function better. Any practicing chiropractor who adjusts people at least twice knows that they go through some very interesting physiological changes. They sleep better, for example, and their quality of life changes because of the adjustment. We also see changes in lifestyle, relationship, and consciousness, attributed to chiropractic care by the patient. This cannot be ignored and must be looked at.

Now the mechanistic side of our profession seeks to keep chiropractic in a musculoskeletal box. It appears to be safe, and as of now, our only research substantiates it.

There almost appears to be a fearful resistance to claiming ownership of our vitalistic roots because there is currently no research. True, our research is very limited and we need much, much more. However, our basis of research needs to expand. Instead of scoffing at the clinical reality of what we are seeing in our practices, the profession needs to get current with the trends in science as they begin to explore, discover, and integrate with the intangible.

Instead of scoffing at the clinical reality of what we are seeing in our practices, the profession needs to get current with the trends in science as they begin to explore, discover, and integrate with the intangible.

Also, as a vitalistic profession, we need to lead other healing professions in our discoveries. Vitalism is not about the treatment and alleviation of symptoms — it is about restoring function and enhancing the human potential. This is the future of chiropractic: leaders in the vitalistic movement — if we have the courage and unity to step up to it.

As more vitalistic types of care are emerging, people are beginning to speak the language. Even MDs and other professionals are talking about innate intelligence, energy flow, and all the things that D.D. and B.J. said way back when. I still do not understand why our profession doesn't "own" its roots in vitalism, especially at this time when the shift is happening around the world. Why would we step behind the movement and allow it to pass us by?

How do chiropractic and performance relate?

I like the word "expression" better than "performance." By improving neurology, we affect all sensory input and function. If we are improving neurological state of function, that's huge in terms of performance. Do we have the literature yet? No. Do we need it? Absolutely.

But we don't need to wait until we see those results published. I can cite, along with many, many practitioners, miracle stories about how people's lives changed under chiropractic care. It's not just in terms of physiology and quality of life either. Their thought patterns and their overall ability to express more life have improved as well. For me, chiropractic is not about health care, it's about the expression of life.

How does chiropractic relate to a person realizing his or her fullest human potential?

We don't even know what our fullest human potential is. We can only know that by experiencing and observing the evolution of that potential. We also know that invasive procedures that are performed from conception throughout childhood have to be impairing neurology. The physical, emotional, and chemical stresses that we are up against daily in our society impair that neurology.

Patients benefit from the adjustments and lifestyle support they receive from their chiropractors, so they can makes choices that are more congruent with expressing a healthier and greater potential in their lives.

How does chiropractic offer people an opportunity to realize an enhanced quality of life?

It helps to redirect them away from looking outside of themselves for the expression and enhancement of life and focus their attention within. When I'm looking outside of myself, I'm coming from a powerless, fear base. "I'm not good enough." "I'm not this enough." "I'm not *that* enough." "I can't, I can't, I can't." What factors outside of me are going to help me be more of me?

Instead, people ought to be asking, "Who am I, really, and how can I express that?" Let me trust in who I am and let me allow myself to live from that place of knowing.

For example, pregnant women tell us they go to the OBGYN and week after week are told, "your blood pressure is too high (or low), your ultrasound isn't normal, we'd better check this." Everything is fear-based, measured against an arbitrary standard that somebody decided is "normal." But that really doesn't apply to each individual person.

When these same women go to a chiropractor, they get adjusted and are put into biomechanical balance. Their physiology improves, their nerve system interference is reduced, and their bodies are allowed to function better. They are introduced to the perspective that the wisdom within them warrants trust and respect. They begin to regain confidence in the natural process of pregnancy and birth.

Birth itself, by its very nature, is going within and trusting that the body knows what it's doing. In working with pregnant moms for 30 years now, I have discovered that there are three contributing factors leading to difficult labor: physical, emotional, and medical stress. The doctor of chiropractic addresses the cause of these three stressors in practice.

Physical stress in pregnancy affects the alignment of the sacrum and pelvis, which directly affects labor. Specific adjustments can rebalance the pelvic muscles and ligaments, restore nerve system function, and contribute to a safer, easier delivery for both the mother and baby.

Emotional stress in pregnancy is rampant just by nature of the hectic lifestyles we are living. Many of us are in a constant fight-flight state and of course this sympathetic override will have a direct effect on the infant's developing neurology and, of course, birth outcome. We know that the adjustment affects her neurology and can alleviate these fight-flight patterns. Additionally, the core philosophy of chiropractic — trusting the inherent wisdom of our bodies — is a huge gift we give our pregnant mothers. She is redirected back to trusting the process. This is a huge factor in avoiding intervention and difficult labors.

The third contributing factor for difficult labor is medical stress. The whole mechanistic/medical model is fear-based and directs women to look for strength outside of themselves rather than within. What we also know from the research is that every single medical intervention leads to further interventions. Each intervention causes greater difficulty in labor.

When a woman goes to a chiropractor, she receives information about birthing not so readily available. This information will expand her knowledge so she can make her own informed choices. Maybe then she'll decide not to get induced. Maybe then she'll speak up and not allow so many ultrasounds to be performed. Maybe then she'll be very cautious about which birth provider and place of birth she chooses.

The family wellness chiropractor provides the woman with names of other vitalistic practitioners in her community who will also support her through her pregnancy and birth process. Empowered by this knowledge and supported by the right team, these women come up to birth with a completely different perspective, with less fear and more trust.

I have worked with pregnant moms now for more than 30 years. I had all six of my children at home, and we actually did the first four ourselves. We had a midwife for the last two. We had our children the way we did because we understood that pregnancy and birth are normal and natural functions, which my body was completely capable of performing.

What do you feel has happened to the chiropractic profession that
may have limited it from being seen by the world in its true nature?

We worked to be accepted by the big monopolies: insurance
companies and the medical profession. By seeking acceptance into their
paradigm we compromised our vitalistic roots. Ironically, vitalism is
coming back now. The public is demanding it and traditional providers
are questioning their own care.

We need to rethink this direction or we're going to miss a huge
opportunity for chiropractic. I speak at midwifery, obstetric, and other
health conferences. At even the most holistic ones, when I speak about
the chiropractic perspective on vitalism, their mouths drop! I'm not
saying we're better than they are, but we have a grasp of vitalism on a
very deep level. We could actually be leading this whole movement,
rather than chasing after acceptance from the dying mechanistic model.

Chiropractic has become tagged as a pain relief specialty. In your
opinion what more does it have to offer people?

It offers the enhancement of nerve system function, which is really
indefinable at this point, even by cutting-edge science. I'm talking
beyond medical science (which isn't cutting-edge science), but the *real*
cutting-edge science that's looking at the nervous system and discovering how the mind, body, and spirit are all connected via the nervous
system. We need to look at true cutting-edge science to substantiate
what we do, rather than rely on the old, limited model.

What is the purpose of the chiropractic adjustment, and how does not
receiving chiropractic care impact one's life?

The purpose of the adjustment is to reduce nerve interference and
bring about the greater expression of life. If you are not getting
adjusted, your expression of life and your ability to function at your
maximum potential is inhibited.

What is your favorite quote, and how has it impacted your life?

In a chiropractic context, I enjoy and most resonate with the one I
mentioned earlier. Years ago, while meditating, these words of wisdom sur-
faced: "We are all beings in a body needing to love and be loved." I feel it
is very relevant to everything we do. Sometimes life seems so hard, but it
really is about expressing and receiving as much love as we are capable of.

That means respect, honor, trust, and opening ourselves to each
other while realizing that everyone comes from their own perspectives
and interpretations. The fact that people have different ideas doesn't

mean they're wrong. They just have their own personal experiences leading to their own personal perspective.

If I say they're completely wrong, I'm not listening to them or loving them. Let me look past their personal perspective, which is learned behavior, and try to see the greater essence of who they really are. The fabric of this essence, the matrix that connects us, is this love. That's all that we need to give and that's all that we need to receive. If we can focus on that, we can be functioning at a higher level of consciousness and therefore contributing to the "raising of the consciousness" — another one of my favorite quotes.

How is chiropractic unique and what does it offer that other health professions do not?

It's unique in that it is vitalistic, and that separates it from typical mechanistic care. Many holistic therapies are only partially practicing from the vitalistic perspective today, even though their roots were completely vitalistic. Homeopathy, for instance, wasn't created for the treatment of disease, yet now people use homeopathy to treat conditions and diseases, the same way acupuncture is used to treat conditions rather than enhance expression. Unfortunately, the mechanistic model is swallowing up these practices.

We are at a critical point where chiropractic may be compromised, as well. I do not look at chiropractic as a natural *treatment* for kids who come in. It's not a natural cure for any condition or disease. That's not what this is about at all. We are not treating; we are enhancing normal body function. It's not just a play on words, it is a completely different base from where we come from. That's what makes the difference.

What do you sense was the intention behind the creation of chiropractic?

Supposedly, it was by accident, but I don't believe there are any accidents or coincidences. However, it probably surprised D.D. Palmer as much as anyone else when he made his adjustment and Harvey Lillard started hearing. He was a type of vitalistic healer prior to that and this experience with Harvey led him to further develop the philosophy.

D.D. recognized it, questioned it, pursued it and moved forward with it. Look at Einstein and Edison and how they invented things. They were doing their work when all of a sudden a spark of inspiration came and they were led in the direction of a major discovery.

Who are some of your mentors and what impact have they had on your life?

In chiropractic, one of my two biggest mentors was Joe Flesia, whom I miss dearly. He didn't get enough credit and recognition for what he did for this profession. He was really the first to explain the effects of the birth process, the insult it can have on the neurological system, and the chiropractic role for correction. He edited the birth trauma video I produced and, when he was passing, he e-mailed me and said, "I'm glad to know that you will carry the torch." I was quite humbled by him saying that to me. Joe was a big mentor for me.

I later met Dr. Larry Webster, who was a pediatric chiropractic expert. At the time, I didn't really understand that there was such a great need to teach practicing chiropractors how to adjust children. I had learned how to adjust children at my school and had been doing so for many years in our practice. I took his classes in pediatric chiropractic out of interest in fellowship with doctors of like mind, and the next thing I knew, I was on the board of his ICPA.

What turns you on creatively, spiritually, or emotionally?

That's three different avenues of getting turned on. My favorite thing in the world is people. I love people. I love meeting people, I love connecting with people, I love communicating with people, and I love sharing important ideas with people.

That in itself turns me on, and when I wake up in the morning, it's the people I am going to interact with that excite me. It's all kind of integrated and I don't know how to define this more specifically for you, but I enjoy life. I am very grateful for this life. My body works very well for me and I drag it all over the world and it willingly complies.

I like getting up in the morning hearing the birds singing their little hearts out and I say, "Wow I'm alive, and I'm still here, and I've got more time to express and see what's going to come this day." In terms of communication, I love how ideas come through and spark more ideas and I particularly enjoy watching visions, and ideas come into manifestation.

Where do you see the profession 10 years from now?

I see chiropractors as the leaders in vitalism, the leaders of family wellness, and an integral part of the lifestyle and health choices for families. That is the only vision I choose to hold, in spite of the insanity that appears to be happening. That is the focus I have — with vitalism, family wellness, and family lifestyle.

What profession other than your own would you like to have attempted?

As a kid, I always knew I was going to be a teacher. Well, I do teach within chiropractic by doing health care classes and teaching in the community. I was also a writer as a kid. Actually, I'm doing the three things that, as a kid, I knew were important: writing, teaching, and chiropractic. Chiropractic has allowed me to do all that I knew I was destined to do.

Are there any other comments you'd like to share about the wonders of chiropractic?

As much as we think we know about chiropractic, we don't know anything. Today, we're on the brink of understanding, as quantum sciences are unfolding perspectives and knowledge well beyond what is considered to be status quo. We are on the brink of whole new era of science. That's where chiropractic is going to find its home and its validity. Since that is such an enormous field and is just being opened up, I don't know what to say except WOW! Let's release our hold on the limited and take the ride!

Years from now, when people look at your tombstone, what would you want them to read?

There won't be a tombstone. Never did understand the concept. Rather, they can look at a picture and see the passion for life in my eyes and know I am loving the new expression of life I will be having.

Since 1981, **Jeanne Ohm, D.C.,** has had a family, wellness-based practice. She is now an international lecturer on chiropractic care in pregnancy and infancy and a post-graduate instructor for numerous chiropractic colleges. In addition, she authored numerous papers on pregnancy, birth, children and chiropractic and produced both the children's chiropractic song "Power On!" and the educational video "Birth Trauma: A Modern Epidemic."

Dr. Ohm is founder of the "Makin' Miracles... Connecting Kids & Chiropractic," community outreach programs and tools to educate children and adults about the chiropractic wellness lifestyle. She also serves as executive coordinator and executive secretary for the International Chiropractic Pediatric Association (ICPA), and editor of the ICPA's quarterly publication.

A member of the board of directors of the Academy of Chiropractic Family Practice and Holistic Pediatric Association, Dr. Ohm also serves on the advisory board for the Foundation for Health Choice and Families for Natural Living, as a panel member of Mothering magazine Ask the Expert, and as executive editor of *Pathways to Family Wellness* magazine.

Tony Palermo

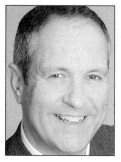

Where are you from originally and what was your childhood like?

I'm originally from Paramus, New Jersey, about 15 miles west of Manhattan. I had a great childhood as an only child. My mom and dad are both business owners and entrepreneurs. My dad, I guess you could say, was my first success coach. Working alongside him, I had the opportunity to learn some great lessons in business. I grew up in what would be considered a charmed life on many levels. I was very well provided for materially and my earliest memories revolve sitting at the kitchen table with mom and dad talking about business. I was a passive participant until I was about 9 years old, but as I grew older I became more and more involved in the conversations about business. So, success has been ingrained in me ever since I was a little kid.

What inspired you to get involved with chiropractic?

I am a prime example of how chiropractic is not necessarily the first choice people make. Unfortunately, in many cases, it's the last resort. Around the age of 18 or 19, when I was an undergrad, I started to suffer from allergies, what the medical profession called "18-year-old allergies."

Now that I sit back and reflect on it all these years later, what a coincidence that I happened to get them at the right age! To make a very long story short, I grew up in a very medically oriented family. If something was wrong you went first to the white-coated family doctor and then to a specialist, which is why I'm a full believer in the concept that specialists are those who know more and more about less and less until they know everything about nothing.

I went to a chiropractor just to shut up my dad's friend, Joe. He kept nagging me, "Go see my chiropractor, go see my chiropractor." I'd already suffered with allergies for about five years at that point and from age 18 to my early 20s endured not only the physical ailments but the side effects of the different medications I was on. I went from being a very active sports enthusiast to the point where running full court in basketball in a pick-up game was literally a life and death situation. I couldn't breathe and was on inhalers and corticosteroids.

My fifth visit and adjustment was literally one of those life-altering situations. My chiropractor, Dr. Larry Nantista, came into the room and asked me how I was doing and I told him I was great. He asked me if I had any questions, and I asked, "How do I do what you're doing for the rest of my life? How do I become a chiropractor?" The words came out of me before there was any real conscious thought. The rest, as they say, is history and I've never looked back. As a kid, I literally loathed science courses yet I excelled in all of the pre-requisite chiropractic classes and on through the chiropractic program as well.

Where do you currently reside and how are you spending your time these days?

I'm on the East Coast of Pennsylvania, in the town of Bethlehem, which is right by the New Jersey border and still close to home. I'm a practicing chiropractor, serving my community for 20-plus years now, and I also serve as a coach in the chiropractic profession, giving 30 presentations a year. I met my beautiful wife in undergraduate school, and we have two beautiful daughters, one is a sophomore in college and the other's a high school senior. This means we're facing the empty nest syndrome in six months, truly the double edged sword of child rearing. On one hand, my wife and I are looking at each other saying, "Wow, check out the freedom!" At the same time, we realize our babies are going to be gone.

How does the profession differ now from when you first became involved?

I would say the number one thing I notice is that there's more global acceptance and our "brand" is recognized. Whether we like the recognition and branding or not, we're more widely accepted and more widely known. The number one television show right now, "Two and a Half Men," features a character named Alan who's a chiropractor. The awareness level about chiropractic has significantly skyrocketed in the past 10 years and definitely in the 27 years I've been involved in it.

Chiropractic was one of those things you went to almost covertly years back. I ask practice members if they'd like me to send periodic updates on my findings to their family medical physician. When I started doing that 15 or so years ago, about half would say, "No, I'd prefer you didn't." Now I find that maybe one in 50 is reluctant to have me contact their M.D., and it's typically a senior citizen who acts almost like he or she would rather keep visits our little secret. People are now far more accepting of chiropractic than they were 20 years ago, and certainly more now than 100 years ago when we first started our game.

How do chiropractic and performance relate?

Chiropractic relates to all aspects of our lives. I tell people it's almost as if we are a brain and a spinal cord and all the rest is just pretty gift-wrapping. For the most part, we're nervous systems experiencing life and therefore everything is translated and processed through the nervous system: performance; overall health and well-being; our relationship to the environment; every aspect of our mental, emotional, physical, chemical, and spiritual lives. We live our lives through our nervous system and interference with the nervous system is like wearing a blindfold when you're driving a car. You wouldn't want to do that, and you wouldn't want to drive your life with a blindfold on your nervous system. If you do, ultimately it's going to wreak some sort of havoc and in chiropractic we define that as dis-ease.

> *I'm a huge fan of finding the extreme in life, in relationships, and in every aspect of life. That's where the real juice is.*

How does chiropractic relate to a person realizing his or her fullest human potential?

The coach and the Socrates inside me always ask, "What is the fullest potential of life?" and "What is one capable of?" For some people, it means just getting through the day, having dinner, watching two hours of television, going to bed, and getting back up to go to work the next day. We can certainly approach and help those individuals to perform better in their day-to-day activities.

On the other side of the coin, there are people who live to the extreme. In fact, I'm a huge fan of finding the extreme in life, in relationships, and in every aspect of life. That's where the real juice is. When you take the blindfold off, all those synapses start firing and our nervous system is going at full speed.

How does chiropractic offer people an opportunity to realize an enhanced quality of life?

Again we have to ask, "What's quality of life?" The more we can interact with life, the greater our experience of life will be. When we're limited, whether it's because of physical ailments or emotional crutches, our quality of life is limited. In enhancing the human potential, we're broadening, widening, and deepening that quality of life.

What do you feel has happened to the chiropractic profession that may have limited it from being seen by the world in its true nature?

I believe that there are two ways to look at this. One of my absolute favorite quotes is, "The present is always perfect and the physical universe never lies." We can live in the past and wonder, "Had we gone this way ..." or we can live in the future and say, "We need to go that way..." Or, we can live in the present and say, "We're living in a time when chiropractic is more widely known and accepted than ever before." I think that the present is perfect right where it is.

> **It may not seem right but if I search deeply enough, dig a little bit, look at it from another angle, maybe heighten my perspective, I can always find 'the perfect' in the situation.**

It may not seem right but if I search deeply enough, dig a little bit, look at it from another angle, maybe heighten my perspective, I can always find "the perfect" in the situation.

Chiropractic has become tagged as a pain relief specialty. In your opinion what more does it have to offer people?

I can speak from my own journey into chiropractic. As I mentioned, I first went to a chiropractor just to shut up my dad's friend. I actually gave my chiropractor a piece of paper listing all the medications I was on. I may not have been typical in that I didn't have back or neck pain, but I went to a chiropractor with symptoms, just like most people do.

The beauty of our profession is its ability to remove the interference to healing. There is such a depth, a breadth of knowledge, consciousness, and wisdom that's available to us as long as we're willing to take the next step to learn more.

What is the purpose of the chiropractic adjustment and how does not receiving chiropractic care impact one's life?

This may sound a bit arrogant but I'm speaking as a chiropractic patient and not as a chiropractor when I say that chiropractic care is a privilege and not a right. It was a privilege that I was referred to, met with, and had my life transformed by the power of an adjustment. It's a privilege to receive a chiropractic adjustment and, for chiropractors, a privilege to deliver a chiropractic adjustment. What's possible as the result of a chiropractic adjustment? Good Lord, the possibilities are infinite.

How is chiropractic unique and what does it have to offer that other health professions do not?

We are unique in our philosophy. Plenty of healing arts have a practice but do not have a philosophy. We have both the philosophy and the practice. We have the sound fundamental science to show that interference with the nervous system does, can, and will cause interference to health. We have scientific proof of that.

We have philosophical proof that when the human body is functioning at 100 percent and there is no interference to the source of life — the nervous system — the body can and does heal. Not only does it heal physical ailments, but spiritual and emotional components as well.

Lastly, we have the art of chiropractic, the adjustment. The adjustment is completely different from an osteopathic manipulation which is grosser in its nature. As B.J. Palmer said about the chiropractic adjustment, "If it is not specific, it is not chiropractic."

We have the best of both worlds. We have a practice and a philosophy. We stand unique because of our philosophy.

What do you sense was the intention behind the creation of chiropractic?

I believe the intention was to find a healing method that would bring relief. From there, I think the real genius was when D.D.'s son, B.J., created a dynamic philosophy that went far beyond just helping people get well, one that truly has the potential to heal the planet without side effects.

Who are some of your mentors and what impact have they had on your life?

My dad, Anthony "Tony" Palermo. Also, Sid Williams and quite a few others along the way have left an impression on me. Dr. Dick Santo, a practitioner from New Jersey, who I think is the spiritual leader of the profession, has had a great impact on my life. Larry Markson definitely was one who taught me how to be a class act. Larry is a gentleman and just simply a class act.

What are some things, if any, that you have had to give up in order to devote your life to chiropractic?

It's the complete opposite. I have gained so much in my life, so many opportunities, so many relationships, so many experiences, that honestly and truly I don't think I've given up anything for it.

Every day, I wake up feeling blessed and thankful for the restoration of my health. I just turned 50 last week and I was reflecting on what would have happened if I hadn't taken this path. What if I'd continued taking the medication I was on and stayed in the strictly medical model seeking the relief of my symptoms? I know for a fact I would be like many of the guys I went to undergraduate school with. When we get together at gatherings, they're all talking about which pills they're taking for what ailment. They look at me and wonder how it's possible that I am still fitting into jeans I wore so long ago and why I'm so healthy. It's directly related to living the chiropractic lifestyle. I eat well, get adjusted regularly, get proper rest, keep my mind free and clear, and do regular exercise.

What turns you on creatively, spiritually, or emotionally?

I've always been a creative type and one of the things I love about chiropractic is the creative aspect of the art of adjusting. I do 30 presentations a year and I spend a lot of time at these events learning more about the art of adjusting. I'm always looking for other ways and methods of delivering a chiropractic adjustment, which totally jazzes me.

I love to write articles and books for the chiropractic profession and for my community. The entire process and field of chiropractic is a complete turn-on to me because it taps into my creativity and it touches my spiritual side. I consider myself, while not very religious, extremely spiritual. Chiropractic taps into my ability to serve humanity. I believe we've been placed on this earth to accumulate knowledge and share it with others. I look for every opportunity to share with those who would like to learn more about themselves, the way their mind works, the way their body works, the human-physical and human-spiritual connection, etc.

A long time ago one of my coaches, Tom Leonard, asked me to define what I do — in 10 words or less! I really struggled with that. My wife says, "Some people are afraid to speak in public, well my husband is afraid to shut up." It took a good six weeks of work to figure out those 10 words, and then he said to cut it down to five! That got really difficult but I got it down to five words. Finally, he said to cut it down to three.

I said to him, "I remove interference," and that was the answer. It just spilled out and it was one of those moments where Innate was working through me. It was an example of Universal Intelligence being translated into my life experience.

Interference of the mind, the nervous system, or the body — whatever is impeding or interfering with an individual's ability to take the next step toward a better quality of life or fulfillment of his or her innate potential; I remove that interference and help the person eliminate it from his or her life completely.

Where do you see the profession 10 years from now?

Chiropractic is going to thrive and prosper in spite of its members and because of its members. Chiropractors at their "soul-ular" level and at their cellular level are complete renegades, lone wolves, and rebels. In spite of how it may appear, we have embarked on a profession that is misunderstood, unknown to many, unfamiliar to most. The onion is big and we have a lot of peeling to do to get to the core of it. Our renegade spirit has the potential to keep us moving forward, thriving, kicking fannies, and taking no prisoners. However, we have to recognize the fact that the lone wolf, individual, and pioneer spirit sometimes gets in the way.

I have absolute faith and conviction that chiropractic will survive. That's why I coach other chiropractors and that's the reason I leave my family behind 30 weekends a year to go on the road and meet, speak with, and teach chiropractors. I received a beautiful e-mail from a chiropractor I met when doing a 10-hour presentation in Austin, Texas. His e-mail was a reminder that there's always hope, the present is always perfect, and the physical universe never lies. The doctor wrote: "I showed up at this event strictly because I needed the CE hours. My intention was to just get through the hours because I had a plan that within the next year to two years maximum, I was out of this profession. For the first time in 17 years as a chiropractor, I understand what my purpose is and I have no intention of quitting and I would like to get in touch with you and have you as my coach, taking the journey together."

Like this doctor, I have no doubt there is a stick-to-it mentality and a tenacity built into chiropractors and we just will not quit. I see bright and beautiful things ahead for our profession.

What profession other than your own would you like to have attempted?

As a result of my involvement in chiropractic, I've been able to truly explore every possible career. A job or a career is something you do in order to have money, a house, your kid's college tuition, and savings. But a vision or a calling is something that you *have* to do.

I've asked myself what careers really jazz and excite me. I came up with playing music and writing. I am a writer in the profession and I still play my music. I've also been involved in political lobbying for chiropractic. I've had several businesses within the chiropractic profession both as a coach and a practicing chiropractor with two clinics. I have really had the opportunity to do anything and everything all while standing firmly on the platform and foundation of chiropractic.

Years from now when people look at your tombstone, what would you want them to read?

He removed interference.

❧

A 1989 Life University graduate, **Tony Palermo, D.C.,** has operated two highly successful chiropractic practices during the past 20 years. His 100% cash, 100% referral-only practice is a model for chiropractors around the world.

Dr. Palermo is a post-graduate, continuing-education faculty member at Life University School of Chiropractic, a past team teacher for the Chiropractic Leadership Alliance's Total Solution, and an author with more than 100 articles published in a variety of chiropractic trade publications. He has spoken before thousands of doctors at chiropractic gatherings, conventions, and seminars worldwide.

In 2003-04, he held the position of CEO of the World Chiropractic Alliance, and was the Chiropractic Leadership Alliance senior vice-president in 2007-08.

Dr. Palermo also serves as a senior partner of the Upper Cervical Health Centers of America with offices located throughout the world. A professionally trained success coach, "Dr. Tony" is an expert in helping professionals create the lifestyle of their dreams.

Guy Riekeman

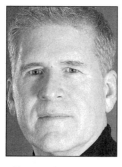

Where are you from originally and what was your childhood like?

My father was a chiropractor and graduated in 1947 from Palmer, moved to Albuquerque, set up an office on 14th and Central Avenue, and started seeing patients when visits were two dollars apiece. There was no insurance, no research, and my mother ran his office. In fact, my mother, at 85, is still running my sister's office. My sister took over for my father when he retired.

Chiropractic historian Dr. Joseph Keating did research on how medical doctors were using state boards to keep chiropractors out of their states. He discovered that my father was the only chiropractor ever appointed by a governor to serve on the medical state board to oversee the pathology portion of the exam for chiropractors and other professionals taking that exam.

In those days, you had to go through the medical basic sciences exam and then take a specialty exam like chiropractic. While they did have a chiropractic board and a chiropractic license in many states, the medics would make sure that chiropractic applicants did not get through the basic science exam to be able to take the chiropractic exam.

Exams consisted of essays back then — no multiple choice or fill in the blanks — so grading was very subjective. My father was placed by the governor on the medical board as the only chiropractor. Dr. Don Kern, the president of Palmer College of Chiropractic, remembers taking the pathology exam from my dad in New Mexico when he was getting his license.

So, I was raised in a chiropractic family. We are now three generations of non-vaccinated and non-drugged human beings. I have a sister who's a chiropractor, and three brothers. My daughter and son-in-law are both chiropractors and practice in Colorado Springs and of course their kids have not been drugged or vaccinated either. In fact, my oldest grandson, Tyler, who is 10 years old, told us that one of the kids in his school was ranting at the teacher and his mother saying, "I wish I was like Tyler so I didn't have to take drugs."

Tell us a little about your Intellectual Board of Trustees.

I designed my Intellectual Board of Trustees as a "think tank" I carry around with me. Every major corporation has a board of directors that provides advice, information, and dialogue about issues facing their business. I thought it would be great if I could have one of those personally for my life issues.

Over a period of time, I began to realize I'd been developing what I call this Intellectual Board of Trustees. I have about 12 people on it and each is there for a specific reason.

One of them is Walter Payton of the Chicago Bears because he ran, over the course of his career, nine miles on the football field. That doesn't sound remarkable except for the fact that he was getting knocked down every three and a half yards by really big, mean guys. Yet he kept getting up.

Yul Brenner, who died of cancer from smoking his whole life, was on my Board of Trustees and he commented one time: "After the final 'no' there is a 'yes' and on that yes the future of the world depends." You can always say no to all of the reasons why something happens but ultimately you have to say yes to health and yes to life and then the direction gets really clear.

B.J. Palmer was on my Board as well. Some members were real-life people and some were fictional. My father was on it because he was a very strong individual but the most quiet, gentle, and kind man I have ever met. I never heard anyone say a thing against him. Yet he was part of a group of chiropractors taking a stand for their profession in Albuquerque. One of their offices was fire-bombed and another had his office ransacked. They all thought that perhaps they should back off for a while but dad spoke up and told them, "No, we are doing the right thing and we are going to continue." They listened to him.

I placed my grandson Tyler on the Board as chairman because of something that occurred at the birth of my second grandson, Caelen. My daughter, Vanessa, wanted everyone at the birth, including Tyler. We decided he shouldn't be there for those last few moments when the head crowns, especially since, at his birth, Vanessa was screaming at the top of her lungs "Get this thing the hell out of me!"

It was my job to have Tyler out of the room at the right moment. We were sitting outside and got the word that Caelen had entered the world. I whisked Tyler into the room. There's an emotion that goes on in those rooms that causes people to collapse, cry, and will even make mean old men break down in tears. I wanted to see what would happen to this 3 1/2-year-old when he walked into the room after the birth of his brother.

He walked into the room and he didn't even see Caelen, who was still hooked to the umbilical cord on Vanessa's stomach. Tyler crawled into bed with Vanessa, placed his arms snugly around her, brushed wet hair out of her face and kissed the back of her hand. We were all just silently amazed at this flow of love coming out of Tyler.

Then he spotted Caelen. He was right there in the bed and didn't even see his brother. His life changed at the moment he saw him. He was going back and forth between Caelen and Vanessa and didn't know which one to give the most attention to when all of a sudden he snapped out of whatever zone he was in, turned to his dad and said, "Well, what is he going to be for Halloween?"

At that moment, he went on the Board because every now and again we get caught up in all this stuff in life and we have to stop and remember what's really important. Tyler reminds me of that.

What inspired you to get involved with chiropractic?

I was an All-American high school basketball player and that's what I wanted to do. I was playing at New Mexico my first year and hated the coach. I decided to transfer to DePaul University in Chicago and play for old man Ray Meyer. You had to sit out a year at the time and it was during the Vietnam War, so you didn't want to be sitting out at home because it was an automatic draft.

My dad said I should go to Palmer because it was close to Chicago and I could go watch the games and, besides, who knows what I'd want to do in the future. I went there and in my third quarter — the classic October-to-June kind of school experience — Dr. Virgil Strang, who was teaching anatomy, said he'd give us extra credit points if we'd listen to some guy speak for four hours one night and four hours the next night in this old, dark, dank auditorium.

At that time of year in Davenport, Iowa, there really isn't that much to do anyway, so a bunch of us decided to go. We walked into the room and three hours into it, I couldn't have told you what was being said, but in retrospect I knew, in that moment, what I was going to do for the rest of my life.

The speaker was Reggie Gold. The only reason I think I could tell you now what he probably said back then is because he's saying the same thing today. We hear it from him over and over and over again and the message is still true.

I was part of a group that met every weekend and we'd stay up all weekend talking philosophy. We'd always look for new "victims" to bring in. We'd find some first-quarter students and get them to come over and ask the questions all fledgling chiropractors had such as, "What about vaccination?" or "What about germs?" From this, we were building our case and answering their questions.

Gerry Clum, who was a little behind me in school at Palmer, started bringing students to the Dynamic Essentials meetings in Atlanta. Mick Hamilton, a chiropractor who practiced in California, and I started producing an underground newspaper at Palmer called the Spinal Column, which was very controversial at the time.

After graduating, I opened up a "Box on the Wall" practice, where people put any amount they could afford for an adjustment in a box. A "Box on the Wall" practice is a more difficult practice to manage because, rather than having a regular fee, you have to make sure you hold people responsible for paying what they can afford. It's based on the notion, of course, that people can't afford health so they're paying for the services, education, time, and the clinic itself.

After two years with the "Box on the Wall" practice, we went to a simple fee upper-cervical Blair Technique practice. The office was based on patient education and the first patient visit consisted of a two and a half hour health care class. People came to that class and, at the end, decided whether or not to be under care.

Where do you currently reside and how are you spending your time these days?

I live in Midtown Atlanta. I also have a ranch in Colorado that's 500 acres in the middle of four million acres of Pike National Forest, so I don't need any more land. I live in a really wonderful place right in downtown Atlanta on the 17th floor with great city views. A mountain ranch and a city condo is perfect balance.

I'm president of Life University, which is 15 minutes away. My time is spent almost exclusively at the college and as a director on the Board of Directors at the Council on Chiropractic Education (CCE).

I travel a great deal because I still do a lot of speaking, almost exclusively for the school. We're doing a "Power of One" tour, hitting 100 cities in two and a half years, bringing the message of chiropractic and how to make lives extraordinary. There's a lot of roadwork and very little time for myself, although I get to go out on a golf course once in a while, or to a concert or sporting event.

I love events. Anything with a gathering of people, you can sign me up. I wouldn't watch a baseball game on TV, but at the end of the day I love to go to Turner Field and watch the Braves.

I still go to six to eight movies a week, which is part of my fantasy and creative life. I usually start that at about 7 p.m. and get done about midnight. It's better than staying home and watching television. I went to film school at UCLA, so I have this great love of film. In 1995, we produced a documentary for the Chiropractic Centennial that aired on national TV.

How does the profession differ now from when you first became involved?

One of the things is obviously standardization of education. The Council on Chiropractic Education came into being when I was in chiropractic school between 1969 and 1972. It has transformed chiropractic in an unbelievable number of ways, some good and some questionable.

The level of education has been elevated and the CCE has leveled the playing field for students enrolling. In the old days, you'd have someone with a high school education and another with a Ph.D. sitting in the same classroom. It makes it tough on instructors because they have to teach to the lowest common denominator. CCE required the upgrading of the facilities and set standards for the type of people teaching courses, which then upped the cost of going to school.

When I went to school we graduated with no debt. I remember how we screamed when they raised tuition at Palmer from $195 to $215 a quarter. Now, students are graduating $130,000 to $150,000 in debt, which brings with it a whole other level of pressure. One difference, then, is the upgrading of the education and the implications that has for chiropractors.

The profession has also gained a lot of political power. I don't think my father would believe the political clout we have today. There's been a huge recognition and acceptance of chiropractic, not necessarily for what we truly do, but we'll go to Washington and the senators will waltz you into their office and talk to you about chiropractic.

We have a staffed office to adjust the senators and representatives on Capitol Hill. I was in Georgia Sen. Johnny Isakson's office and a staff member who worked there told me: "We can't go and get adjusted because it's only for the senators and congress members. We need an office up here." I told her to get me the space and I'd get her the chiropractor to take care of the staff. That never would have happened in my father's lifetime.

How do chiropractic and performance relate?

On a biological level you can't have performance if you have interference to the nervous system, since the nervous system carries on a dialogue with itself, the body and its environment.

You can't have internal performance — health — if the nervous system isn't working right, and you cannot have normal adaptation to the environment if the nerve system is not carrying on that dialogue with the environment effectively.

We now know, based on Bruce Lipton's work, that that dialogue programs the genes from the time you're born throughout your lifetime. If you're not having an appropriate dialogue because of "cloudiness" in the nerve system, the gene programming is inaccurate and can affect offspring and all sorts of things.

> **On a biological level you can't have performance if you have interference to the nervous system, since the nervous system carries on a dialogue with itself, the body and its environment.**

When they hear the word "performance," most people think of athletic performance. At Life University, we take a broader view of it than that. We have something called the Wellness Portfolio, which includes six "buckets" of performance: physical, emotional, spiritual, intellectual, social, and environmental.

We have created a definition of health and wellness and everything we do at the institution is analyzed in the context of those six buckets. A student coming on campus now fills out an extensive questionnaire which has to do with these six buckets.

Advisors then sit down with the students and find out what their goals are while they're here, relative to those six buckets. We're designing a system to check with them regularly throughout their curriculum to see how they're meeting those goals.

We're moving into new student housing and we have six "Visioneer Groups" that each tackle one category. I'm on the Environmental Visioneering Group. We get together and talk about the new student housing and develop a vision of what it would need to be in order to fit perfectly with the environment. The Social Visioneering Group meets and talks about the people who are going to interact in this environment, and how we can build something that creates wellness through social interaction. Each group comes up with programs, ideas, and structures and then we give that to the architects and the architects design the buildings. When we talk about performance, that's what we mean.

How does chiropractic relate to a person realizing his or her fullest human potential?

When Joe Flesia and I we were doing the Renaissance seminars for years, and then Quest, we talked about potential and called it "The Predicament of the Species." This was back in the '70s, before anyone was talking about predicament of the environment, predicament of the species, or overpopulation. We were thought to be wackos at the time, but it turns out we were the prophets.

One of things we talked about was human potential. The easiest way I can describe it is that we structured our seminars around a metaphor called "the magical child," based on Joseph Chilton Pearce's book of the same name.

Pearce was an anthropologist and he said that a human being goes through a series of what I am going to call "genetic windows." These windows open up for a period of time. In these genetic windows, there needs to be a degree of physical, spiritual, intellectual, relational, emotional, and academic development. Then, the window closes. If you didn't have complete development in all of those areas, the possibilities available in the next stage of development are decreased.

If you do not have complete development in the next stage — which you probably won't — then that window closes and the next stage of development is even more limited.

The magical child was a theoretical person who realized full development in all of these areas — physical, spiritual, intellectual, relational, emotional, and academic — at each one of these genetic windows.

A perfect example of this is fertilization. We know that around week five, a fetus' arms and legs begin to develop and within just a few weeks, that stage is done. In the '60s, a drug called Thalidomide was given to women for morning sickness. Because of the effect of this drug, science finally realized that anything that goes into the mother's body goes through the placental barrier and affects the child.

Thalidomide stopped whatever was developing on that day. If it was taken at week six, the child might be born with a flipper instead of an arm or leg. You cannot reach age 40 and decide you're tired of these flippers and want to grow an arm. That stage of development has to occur within a certain genetic window, or it is not going to occur.

To us, optimum performance and optimum potential can be achieved by making sure people develop fully in each one of these windows throughout the entire course of their lifetime.

To do that, first you have to get rid of the interferences like Thalidomide or subluxations that would interfere with proper development. Second, we have to have a consciousness that this is what we want to accomplish and we're not even looking at it, right? The new health care discussion is only about access and cost. They are not talking about a different goal for health care.

Third, we have to create resource-rich environments so when organisms are ready to develop in these areas at certain times, all of the resources they need for development are there.

Children in a Montessori school, for example, may want to spend all day pouring sand back and forth between two cans because that's what they're learning that day. When they need to learn that innately, you have to make sure that the two cans and the sand are there. That is our idea of optimum potential.

How does chiropractic offer people an opportunity to realize an enhanced quality of life?

It goes right back to what we just talked about. First, on a clinical level it removes a major interference — if not THE major interference — to the normal function of the organism and its dialogue with the environment. Secondly, it educates people about greater potential and possibility instead of just getting through life without pain. And thirdly, chiropractic is supportive of other organizations and other vitalistic philosophies that help create the resources people need in order to maximize their potential. For these reasons, we ought to be the gatekeepers into the health care system.

What do you feel has happened to the chiropractic profession that may have limited it from being seen by the world in its true nature?

Money, recognition, and acceptance. But those are classic antagonist and protagonist stories throughout the history of humanity.

There's a Ph.D. from Boston University, Bill O'Brien, who's married to a chiropractor and served on our Life Board of Trustees. He's one of those geniuses who owns a company that does futuristic predicting for Microsoft and other companies that want to know where they'll be in five years and 10 years.

He wrote his thesis on how movements rise and fall, how they come from a purist idea and then, for acceptance, give up certain pieces of that idea. Eventually they give up so much that the idea no longer can be found and the movement dies out.

His thesis focused on chiropractic and traced where our profession was from D.D. Palmer to B.J. and where it is today. His conclusion was that, today, you can hardly tell the difference between a chiropractor, osteopath, or a physical therapist in some cases. We have given up so much of our basic principles and think the answer lies in adding more "stuff" to the pot.

Has adding more "stuff" to the pot of chiropractic clouded the public's perception of chiropractic or aided it positively in some way?

There's no question that it tends to cloud it. There are, however, needed services that chiropractors provide that other people are not providing. I have a good friend who teaches a chiropractic technique class. He is a Gonstead genius practitioner and instructor. He said that while manipulating an extremity — shoulder, wrist, elbow, etc. — is not what he would call chiropractic, no one else can do it. I'm not opposed to chiropractors doing other things, as long as there is clarity of purpose for the patient.

There are certain common areas of general information that all health care practitioners incorporate in their practices. For example, you can direct people to good nutrition whether you're a medical doctor, osteopath, chiropractor, or physical therapist. Same thing with stress reduction, exercise, basic rehabilitation of injuries, etc.

Many chiropractors use varying levels of physical therapy, but what we do in chiropractic isn't really physical therapy, even though we sometimes call it that. It's active rehabilitation with a patient who has injuries related to chiropractic.

Do you feel that chiropractors ought to be administering certain therapies and selling certain nutrition and other products in their office?

I can't comment on what they ought to have and not have in their offices. I can tell you that if it were my office, I would have a neurological focus and chiropractic adjusting of the spine to correct subluxations along with the recognition that people need a resource-rich environment for getting better, maintaining health, and optimizing potential. I would direct my patients to other practitioners for yoga, nutrition, physical therapy, etc.

If you had a chiropractic office today would you have a cash-only practice or would you incorporate health insurance reimbursement?

If patients pay for a health insurance policy and if I don't have to alter what I do to provide optimum health care in order for them to capitalize on this benefit, I'm not opposed to it. I am opposed to it when it limits the practice I have.

I was in Northern Europe with Joe Flesia a number of years ago and we were lecturing about lifetime care to a brick wall. One of the practitioners pulled us aside during the break and said, "You have to understand that in Norway, the Patient Visit Average (PVA) is five visits." We found out later that's how many visits the government paid for. That is unethical.

Chiropractic has become tagged as a pain relief specialty. In your opinion, what more does it have to offer people?

We sold it that way. The pain thing is irrelevant to me. Pain anywhere in the body is just a sign that something is wrong. It's nothing more than a clinical indicator that there is an issue somewhere and we ought to be looking into the body.

If the elimination of the pain is the ultimate outcome, you have to decide whether the patient should be in chiropractic, somewhere else, or some combination. I understand we have to address pain as part of the initial intensive care. For the rest — optimizing function and adaptation of an organism and maximizing potential — there's no health care coverage and I cannot foresee there being any in the near future.

In order for the general public to recognize that chiropractic has more to offer than just the relief of neck and back pain, we have to have a head space shift ourselves. We've convinced ourselves that people are not going to listen to us and we can't tell them what chiropractic is and have them understand it. We began using bizarre terms like joint dysfunction and manipulation instead of subluxation and adjustment, thinking that somehow we could engage them by using their lexicon.

Physical therapists convinced Medicare that they can perform manipulations of joint dysfunction and, all of a sudden, we want to switch back to subluxation and adjustment to distinguish ourselves.

Most chiropractors see themselves as spine specialists and I think that is the least important part of what we do. We are neurologists. If there was no section in the Yellow Pages for "Chiropractor," and we had to choose between "Orthopedics" and "Neurology," we'd have to choose "Neurology." That is what we do. Yet, DCs are putting pictures of spines on their business cards when they should be getting people to understand neurology.

When we give an adjustment, we may not be so much moving a bone as we are stimulating the nerve system. I realize that's oversimplified. If you take a cadaver, you can't move a bone. This only happens in living beings that are having neurological adaptations to the environment. There is a lot of compelling information today that even when we're working on the spine, we are impacting the nerve system.

As a profession, we need to have an agreement on our basic parameters. Several years ago, Dr. David Koch and I came up with seven points. Four of the major ones are now being used by states to enlist their state associations to work together on unity issues.

If we can agree on these four points we ought to move forward. The four points are: 1) the nerve system is central to health and chiropractic, 2) the spine is related to nerve system function, 3) chiropractic has broader ramifications than just getting rid of back and neck pain — it focuses on the correction of spinal malfunction via subluxation correction, and 4) subluxations shouldn't be corrected only when there is symptomatology but whenever they exist throughout one's lifetime.

All chiropractic state organizations in Georgia signed on to this concept. Some doctors may do nutrition and some may just adjust the Atlas only, but all of them said that these four things are absolutely the basis of chiropractic. The Georgia law hasn't been changed since 1921 but all of the organizations got together and now these components — nerve, spine, subluxation, and regular care — are part of the law in Georgia.

What is the purpose of the chiropractic adjustment and how does not receiving chiropractic care impact one's life?

The purpose of the adjustment is to correct the subluxation, which then allows the body to normalize itself and normalize its relationship and dialogue with the environment. That is its purpose. Along the way, pain may go away and a liver may get better, etc.

Those who are not under chiropractic care are going to have a reduced internal dialogue, a reduced dialogue with their environment, which shows up as emotional, physical, social, spiritual, and environmental dysfunctions that at some point may be diagnosed and treated. Ultimately, and through regular chiropractic care, you have to create this normal dialogue.

What is your favorite quote and how has it impacted your life?

I'll give you a couple of them. B.J. Palmer's "Get the big idea and all else follows," is a classic, along with "There is nothing more powerful than an idea which has met its time."

I have a new one from a book "The 4-Hour Workweek," written by Tim Ferriss: "Most people aren't lucky enough to get fired and so they die a slow spiritual death over 30 or 40 years of tolerating mediocrity."

Who are some of your mentors and what impact have they had on your life?

Obviously, Reggie Gold was one of the first ones. A program I took a while back called EST with Werner Erhard made a huge impact on my life. Ayn Rand, the philosopher and writer who wrote "Atlas Shrugged" also had a great impact on my life.

Joe Flesia was certainly a mentor of mine and when I became president of these colleges, Fred Barge worked for me and he was a huge mentor without knowing it. He was fabulous. He came in the first day I hired him and said, "Mr. President, what shall you have me do?" I said to him, "Fred, there are two things I want you to do. I want you to 'Palmerize' Palmer and I want you to walk around and be Fred Barge."

Every morning when I walked into the office he'd be there within five minutes and ask, "Mr. President, what shall you have me do today?" He would start every class he taught with, "Good morning, fledgling chiropractors." One of my favorite quotes was when Fred needed to end his lectures, he simply threw up an overhead which read "enuf said!"

What are some things, if any, you have had to give up in order to devote your life to chiropractic?

Marriage and being home for my kids on so many weekends. In one of his poems, Yeats says: "Man has to choose between labor and love. If he chooses labor, he will leave people screaming in the dark." I have left a lot of people, family, children, and friends screaming in the dark. There's no question about that. Then, you give up being president of Coke which is a much easier job than being president of a university. It is much less political and I think that guy got 20 million last year. They pay me well at Life for being president but not like that.

What turns you on creatively, spiritually, or emotionally?

To put a group of people in a room and see them create something that would not have existed if that group had not been together. That does it for me and gets my juices going for a long time. Sitting in movies gets my juices going. Anything that has to do with art, creativity and a broader expression of the human experience.

In my lecture called "The Seven Disciplines of Excellence," I show a video clip to illustrate each of the disciplines. I show a video clip of Tiger Woods being interviewed by Ed Bradley and one of Yanni directing an orchestra at the Acropolis, where two violin players start inspiring each other and feeding off each other to create a zone of excellence.

I show a clip from a 1950s movie of Fred Astaire and Eleanor Powell doing a tap dance and it's phenomenal how in sync they are. There are many things outside of chiropractic — in sports, business, industry and the arts — that illustrate the releasing of human potential. That's what turns me on.

Where do you see the profession 10 years from now?

People ask me that all of the time. I have no idea. We think in the old mechanistic view that the future can be predicted because it's an extension of the past. What quantum dynamics has taught us is that if you change one critical variable in the system, the outcome is entirely different and usually unpredictable.

I have great hope for the profession, for humanity, and for the environment. The human element changes everything and you cannot predict what the human element and our changing consciousness will do.

What profession other than your own would you like to have attempted?

If I weren't doing this, I'd probably want to be an architect. I don't necessarily like the details involved, but I do like the creativity of envisioning buildings and making something dramatic come out of nothing.

Are there any other comments you'd like to share about the wonders of chiropractic?

We have moved towards wellness care and in doing so left behind the great miracles that come out of chiropractic. People who have tried everything and are on their death beds have come to a chiropractor and regained their health. I would just caution us not to lose sight of the whole spectrum of chiropractic. When we give an adjustment, the entire organism goes into a higher state of vibration, energy, excellence, and optimization of potential and intention and out of all of these elements a different human being is born. Sometimes that shows up as the healing of ulcers and cancers.

At a seminar in St. Louis, a woman in her 80s sat in the front row. She was a most beautiful woman, with such energy radiating from her that I thought she was 50 or 60 years old. She was supposed to die 80+ years ago — at the age of 2. They gave her no hope whatsoever for survival and her distraught father went to see his minister and asked, "What does it mean in the Bible where it talks about the laying on of hands?"

The minister, not knowing what to tell him, said, "I think you should maybe take her to a chiropractor." The woman said her earliest memory as a child was riding the trolley across St. Louis to get adjusted by a chiropractor. In her early 20s, the medics told her she would never be able to get pregnant. She said to them, "I'm going back to my chiropractor."

She pulled out her wallet that night, right there at the seminar, and showed me all of the pictures of her kids and grandkids. "I've been going to a chiropractor once a week for 80-something years," she told me. To me, that's the whole spectrum. We took someone off her death bed and allowed her to realize her dream to have children and then we took care of her and them for lifetime wellness care.

Years from now when people look at your tombstone, what would you want them to read?

"He laid a stone for humanity." Not the final one and not the first one. Simply, "He laid a stone for humanity."

ॐ

Guy F. Riekeman, D.C., the fourth president of Life University, obtained his chiropractic degree with honors in 1972 from Palmer College of Chiropractic. He established a successful practice in Kansas City where he pioneered educational programs to empower patients to be responsible for their own health choices. He worked with Peter Graves, Lorne Greene, Tony Franciosa, Deepak Chopra and others to produce the first-ever health care educational programs videos.

As a leader for the chiropractic centennial celebration in 1995 he produced the nationally aired TV documentary, "From Simple Beginnings," to help inform the public and gain a greater appreciation for chiropractic's contributions to health and wellness.

A successful businessman, Dr. Riekeman created companies and seminar programs to improve chiropractic practice and facilitate personal growth. Quest, founded in 1987, became one of the most widely acclaimed of such professional enterprises. He continues to be highly sought after as a motivational speaker, making dozens of appearances each year before a variety of international audiences.

Terry A. Rondberg

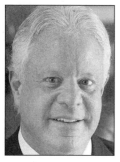

Where are you from originally and what was your childhood like?

I was born in 1951 in St. Louis where my father was born. My mother was born in a little town in Eaton, Ohio. The Navy sent my father to the University of Miami in Ohio before sending him to Harvard for his officer training. He and my mom met on campus, moved back to St. Louis and proceeded to have my older sister, me, and my younger brother. They raised us in a very typical post-WWII middle class suburban experience. My father was fairly successful as a developer and I always thought I was going to go into the development and real estate business with him.

What inspired you to get involved with chiropractic?

My mother went to a chiropractor because she was having severe low back pain and the orthopedic doctors recommended surgery. She wanted to avoid that so she found chiropractic. Our background was Jewish and we didn't even know what chiropractic was. When I was 19 and an undergraduate, I visited my parents for the weekend and had a talk with my mom. She told me she'd been visiting a chiropractor while I was away at school and didn't need surgery now. She told me that it might be a really interesting profession for me to look into.

I asked her what chiropractic was and she explained that a chiropractor was a doctor but a different kind of doctor. She said chiropractors didn't use drugs or surgery and I thought it sounded interesting. I still didn't have any idea what she was talking about but I was ecstatic that she didn't need to go under the knife.

That afternoon, I went with her to her chiropractor, Roy Hilgartner (who ended up being my professor at Logan College of Chiropractic).

He was this young, cool married guy who explained chiropractic to me and I was impressed by the whole thing. I also remember going out to lunch with his business partner at a nice country club he belonged to in St. Louis. He had five brothers who were also chiropractors, and a sister, and their father was a graduate of Palmer Chiropractic College.

I was very impressed by those doctors and the whole experience. I was excited about going into chiropractic even though I wasn't really sure what it all meant yet. But they were excited about what they were doing and their enthusiasm was infectious. I realized, from what they told me, that chiropractic was not mainstream and that there were issues between the professions.

What were some early challenges you faced?

My first experience of discrimination occurred before I even entered into the chiropractic program. I was finishing up some undergraduate hours and went to visit my uncle Max who was a renowned ophthalmologist and on staff as a professor of Washington University.

He had a very busy clinic and I went to him for a routine eye checkup. Although about 12 people were already in the waiting room when I got there, they took me first and I assumed it was because I was a relative. Well, he took me into the exam room, closed the door behind him, sat down and said, "I want to talk to you." He was real serious all of a sudden.

He started talking about how he heard from my mom that I was considering a career in chiropractic medicine. I told him I wasn't sure that's what they called it but that I was indeed interested and I was planning on going into it. He said I shouldn't sell myself short and that if I wanted a career in medicine he could certainly recommend and probably get me into Washington University's medical school because he was a tenured professor there. He thought I was making a huge mistake! He had no respect for the chiropractic profession and gave me the usual warnings, telling me what a poor choice he thought I was making for a career.

I love my uncle Max and have great respect for him but as a child of the '60s, I was very rebellious, against the war, had very long hair, and an overall distrust of the status quo. My uncle was certainly ringing the wrong bell. He was talking to the wrong guy at the right time. He pushed me even farther in the direction I was going. I was even more excited at that point, sitting there with him in that office, than before. It made me feel even more aligned with the chiropractic profession because they were an underdog, an alternative, and that was very appealing to me on many different levels and in various ways, including spiritually.

Where do you currently reside and how are you spending your time these days?

My home is in Rancho Santa Fe, California, which is on the coast just behind Del Mar in San Diego County. I spend most of my time on *The Chiropractic Journal* newspaper, with the Chiropractic Benefit Services malpractice insurance company, and I'm writing two books right now. I've already written five books and these will be the first ones that are not specifically about chiropractic. I'm planning to publish them within the next year. I spend a lot of time writing, at the Yoga studio, paddle boarding in the ocean, weight training, meditating, and walking a lot on the beach. I spend my time enjoying life to the max.

I love spending time with my kids and even more than that, with my three grandchildren. I have also entered into some areas I feel are related to wellness care and are outside of chiropractic. I promote a nutritional drink called Zrii and now I'm also promoting something I am very excited about called iLearningGlobal, which has partnered with 52 of the top 100 speakers in the country.

How does the profession differ now from when you first became involved?

I've been a part of a lot of these changes and many of the differences are a direct result of what we've done in the World Chiropractic Alliance (WCA), which I founded in 1989.

The profession has made great positive shifts and some that are not so positive. Some of the changes I've been able to influence concern the Council on Chiropractic Practice and the guidelines we developed as a team. Those guidelines have just been accepted for a third renewal and are renewed every five years. They are truly the best guidelines and the only subluxation-based guidelines that have been accepted by the National Guideline Clearinghouse, which is our federal government's website for evidence-based guidelines.

I was able to fund the development of those guidelines through Chiropractic Benefits Services, our malpractice insurance company. We use those guidelines to defend doctors who are accused of malpractice for practicing subluxation-based chiropractic. They have been very effective and used all over the world even where we don't have any insureds.

I am also very proud of *JVSR* — *the Journal of Vertebral Subluxation Research*. It is still the largest repository of research involving subluxation but we have mountains to climb in that area. I put a lot of time and energy into chiropractic research and urging doctors to collect data to help us develop the credibility we need and will receive only from huge studies on outcome.

There has certainly been a shift in that there are people in the profession who want to take it in a different direction, wanting it to become more medical. They're still encouraging full-body diagnosis and institutionalizing chiropractic into some form of physical therapy and they'd like to see us almost as physiatrists or osteopaths treating musculoskeletal conditions.

These people have even attempted, through the Council on Chiropractic Education, to redefine the paradigm developed by the Association of Chiropractic Colleges (ACC) by removing the neural component from the definition of the subluxation. That, to me, would be the end of the chiropractic profession. We were able to stop that. To emphasize the neural component is to emphasize the philosophy and the practice objective as B.J. Palmer handed it down to us as a "Sacred Trust." My goal has always been to protect that paradigm, not excluding other paradigms, but to protect that paradigm as the purest form of chiropractic.

How do chiropractic and performance relate?

The very definition of chiropractic includes the word performance. We have improved function, improved performance, an enhanced immune system, and a higher quality of life. Those are the benefits of chiropractic and the ultimate objective of receiving care on a regular basis over a lifetime. I refer to chiropractic as a lifetime, subluxation-based, family wellness care model.

How does chiropractic relate to a person realizing his or her fullest human potential?

Chiropractic is the cornerstone of wellness care. It plays a vital role because wellness care is about a complete experience of consciousness encompassing body, mind, and spirit. It is an integration of those three components which express a higher consciousness, higher quality of life, and the ultimate expression of optimum health. Anything we can do to remove interference, correct interference, and allow the innate wisdom that flows from above, down, inside, out to more fully express itself, allows the human being to have a healthier experience on the planet in a human body.

How does chiropractic offer people the opportunity to realize an enhanced quality of life?

I published the largest study ever completed on quality of life and its effects on 2,800 different patients to date. It was conducted by Dr.

Robert Blanks, a real pioneer in quality-of-life outcome measurements. He currently serves as a dean at Miami University's Medical School.

Dr. Blanks worked with Dr. Donald Epstein several years ago and I published the study in JVSR. It was an incredible study and in a very simple fashion proved that the more people receive chiropractic care, the better they get and the better they perceive their own health to be — and there is no ceiling on the improvements they can achieve!

A self-reported quality-of-life study, which we refer to as a SRQOL, is a subjective measurement tool that determines changes in people's outlook and perception of their own health. It's a gold standard in medicine and is used in hospitals and public health departments all over the world. It's fairly new as far as tests go.

Our profession needs to combine the best quality-of-life studies with the best objective studies that can measure outcome in other ways. We now have tools to measure that and I've been promoting one which is the NeuroInfiniti. It's something that measures life support systems: brain activity, heart activity, etc., on several different physiological components at the same time. We're able to see what happens before and after an adjustment or do comparisons every three months. Those kinds of tests and comparison studies, integrated with the quality-of-life study, are the strongest possible evidence that humanity benefits by receiving lifetime, subluxation-based corrective care.

What do you feel has happened to the chiropractic profession that may have limited it from being seen by the world in its true nature?

The political arm of medicine is the biggest thing that limited the population from receiving care and from understanding what chiropractic is about. That has been by far the biggest adversary we have had and I think the pharmaceutical industry is certainly tied into that to protect its turf because M.D.s are the drug pushers for the drug companies. They have a competing product and their product is medicine.

Whether we like it or not, medicine has made incredible strides in understanding the microcosmic aspects of cells, DNA, disease, and it's all very fascinating. They also perform miracles on a daily basis, which are exaggerated on TV show after TV show. There are certainly miracles involved with skin grafts, plastic surgery, and emergency situations where lives are saved.

Because of the small good that comes from medicine, they've acquired a positive image. They cultivate that image by sending out press releases every day announcing some new discovery they've made or some new disease they'll be able to cure. I refer to this as The Medical

Machine. Even with all the millions raised for Jerry's Kids, there is still no cure for muscular dystrophy. Nor is there for cancer.

According to our federal government, modern medicine is the leading cause of preventable death. According to the WHO last year, the U.S. was ranked only 37th in the list of healthiest nations of the world. Seven out of 10 adults over the age of 40 living in the United States have a chronic degenerative disease.

When I look at those statistics, I see how the medical miracles pale in comparison with the killing of healthy people in our society through the overuse and abuse of intervention, which was designed to save lives and be utilized in emergency situations. It's sickness and disease care being applied to a society that doesn't need 90 percent of it. That kind of "care" makes them sicker and speeds up their deaths. Several million people go to the hospital every year not only for iatrogenic disease but for unnecessary surgeries and procedures, which lead to death. Hundreds of thousands of people die every year from medical mistakes that never should have been made.

How can we change that? If we want a real paradigm shift and see our culture change, we need to do massive studies on large populations showing the effects of regular chiropractic adjustments. When people get adjusted, they get healthier, need fewer drugs, and certainly need less surgery. We can show the savings on a large scale and we could completely reverse the trend of bankrupting our country to pay the higher costs of medicine, most of which are unnecessary.

Chiropractic has become tagged as a pain relief specialty. In your opinion what more does it have to offer people?

First of all, I am very opposed to describing chiropractic as any type of pain relieving procedure or profession. I think our practice objective is quite clear: we are for wellness care rather than disease treatment or pain prevention. That is what medicine's paradigm is for.

Our real paradigm should be focused on how to maximize the innate health potential of every human being. That occurs by people having their spines checked on a regular basis and allowing the expression of Innate at the highest level possible.

I'm not suggesting that we don't need medical procedures, operations, and medicine at times because we do and they save lives. But if people were under chiropractic care, they would not need most of the medical procedures they routinely get first.

If you don't know any better, the first thing you are going to do is go to your medical doctor and get a drug. If that doesn't work, you may resort to surgery or stronger drugs, without ever asking the most obvious question, which is, "What is causing the problem and how do I correct it?"

The answers to that question will often allow for the avoidable poisoning of the body or use of invasive procedures, which can be very incongruent with the body's homeostasis. When you try to cure the body by controlling its physiology, it reacts and those reactions often lead to sickness, disease, hospital visits, and death. That's why I wrote the book in 1993 called "Chiropractic First."

We need to conduct studies based on massive collections of data that prove the advantages and benefits of chiropractic care. We need to take those studies and show the world how people are benefiting, how their function is improving, how their performance is improving, and how their quality of life is enhanced. We need to get all of these studies in *JAMA, the New England Journal of Medicine,* and other prestigious journals. After that, we'll see it in Time, Newsweek, and the popular press at

Our real paradigm should be focused on how to maximize the innate health potential of every human being. That occurs by people having their spines checked on a regular basis and allowing the expression of Innate at the highest level possible.

large. It will go on Oprah, Larry King, and the popular media.

I'll tell you how I'll know when we have arrived: when the average soccer mom is driving down the street with a van full of kids and she looks at her watch and says, "Oh my gosh, it's time to take the kids to the chiropractor for their weekly spinal hygiene check up."

Anything short of that is a sellout. Chiropractors who limit their practice to neck aches, workers comp, PI, and the like because they pay well, but aren't willing to educate the public about chiropractic or contribute to research, aren't making any real contribution.

When I was speaking at a Parker seminar, I asked the attendees (mostly chiropractors) to raise their hands if they had ever seen a miracle in their office. They all raised their hands. I then asked the same group to raise their hands if they had published their miracle in a scientific, peer-reviewed journal. Every hand in the room went down. That's why people look at us like third-rate medicine. It is because we haven't proven ourselves.

In this day and age, if we want to expand beyond the politics of medicine and reach the masses in the large public arena, we need to have overwhelming mountains of data that will convince average people they're much better off going to a chiropractor and getting regular care than risking the treatment of symptoms, conditions, and diseases. That's proactive, it's what we need to do, and it's what I am going to spend the rest of my life trying to do for this profession.

What is the purpose of the chiropractic adjustment and how does not receiving chiropractic care impact one's life?

Not receiving chiropractic care is like playing Russian Roulette. You have no idea if you're subluxated; if there's any type of interference to the expression of life in your body. You certainly have a chance of not being whole, and so it's a huge risk. Your possibility of becoming something less than whole, of breaking down and having a disease or malfunction on some life support system is much greater because you have no way of knowing if you're going to be a victim. If you go in for regular chiropractic care you certainly reduce that risk and you can live a much healthier life.

What is your favorite quote and how has it impacted your life?

Because of my love for chiropractic, most of my favorite quotes are from the *Green Books,* written by B.J., and other things he said, which I routinely publish in my newspaper. B.J. had so many quotes that have inspired me. There is one I memorized from Volume 37 of the *Green Books,* called "The Glory of Going On." His last written words about his sacred trust are the most inspirational I've ever read. Next to that, he wrote a section in 1961 that reads: "With each of us doing our bit, sharing the load, helping to carry the burden, getting into the harness and putting our shoulders to the wheel, putting everything we've got into it, we can and will save chiropractic in its purity for posterity, for rights of the sick to get well with pure unadulterated by hand only chiropractic." That has certainly inspired me, and I'm sure many others, through the years.

What do you sense was the intention behind the creation of chiropractic?

Medicine was pretty scary in the late 1800s; they were using some pretty bizarre treatment methods to try to help people. I think B.J. Palmer, and his father before him, recognized that was a very dangerous road to go down and that there was a more natural way to accomplish increased health in human beings. I think they stumbled across one of the greatest secrets of humanity, which is the ability to restore the communication and unite the spiritual part of the human being with the physical part by giving an adjustment.

Who are some of your mentors and what impact have they had on your life?

Obviously, I didn't know him when he was living (although we were alive at the same time for a while, at least 10 years) yet the greatest mentor in my professional life has been B.J. Palmer. In addition to B.J., I've really enjoyed reading a lot of spiritual books and I read a lot from all different religions. As far as specific mentors, I would say that Thom Gelardi ranks up at the top with Reggie Gold, Joe Flesia, and Sid Williams, all of whom had a significant influence on my early years in the profession. From politics to philosophy, these doctors were the real teachers for me.

What are some things if any, you have had to give up in order to devote your life to chiropractic?

I've gotten so much back from my commitment to chiropractic, I don't feel there have been any sacrifices. I *have* made sacrifices in my life for chiropractic, but not in the way that we ordinarily think about giving up certain things.

What turns you on creatively, spiritually, or emotionally?

I'll tell you what did it for me because I am real clear on this and I've had a lot of time to reflect and think about this over the years. In 1964, when I was a young boy of 13, my parents took me to Temple in St. Louis. They told me there was going to be a very large crowd because a famous speaker was coming who was making rounds across the country and giving speeches on civil rights.

We went as a family and I recall we sat very close to the front row among a crowd of nearly 10,000 people. I was within 10 feet of the Rev. Martin Luther King, Jr., when he gave a speech about his dream. The clarity of that experience is still astounding. I can remember listening to his passionate words about men being created equal by God, and his dream to see society accept all men as being created equal. I took that to heart in much the same way as I did B.J. Palmer's last written words, which I took very personally.

When B.J. told us to protect this sacred trust and guard it well, I felt like he was talking to me and I still do to this day. Whenever I give a talk somewhere, if I have a copy of my book with me, which I often carry just for this purpose, I read his last written words to the audience. It's become a tradition with me because I feel he inspired me, mentored me my whole career, and I want everyone to hear those words.

Where do you see the profession 10 years from now?

The profession is continually on a collision course with itself and down the road I can only hope, pray, and work towards the peaceful resolution of our differences. I started the WCA in 1989 with the hope that the various camps could enjoy mutual coexistence, respect each other, and share a "live and let live" philosophy instead of trying to tear each other down.

Our emphasis is to enhance wholeness, wellness, and allow people to reach optimum potential and their own personal evolution. I do think there's room for everyone.

Unfortunately, "the other side" — and I lovingly refer to the ACA and its political leaders as the Anti Chiropractic Association — has been quite vicious in its attempt to destroy our paradigm. While they've been unable to do it, they have managed to hurt the growth of the pure side of chiropractic by spending hundreds of thousands of dollars of our profession's money to eliminate SCASA, which was a federally approved and recognized accrediting agency for straight chiropractic. There's been great effort and energy expended to push chiropractic into a very medical type of profession with a medical practice objective of treating symptoms, conditions, and diseases.

On the other side of the spectrum, our emphasis is to enhance wholeness, wellness, and allow people to reach optimum potential and their own personal evolution. I do think there's room for everyone. I loved the ACC paradigm when it came out and our organization was the first to publicly endorse it.

We need to focus less on what's wrong with each other and more on what's right about chiropractic. The ACC paradigm summarizes it better than any document I've seen. It defines chiropractic, the subluxation, Innate Intelligence, and our role as a health care profession, and I believe that 10 years from now, if we can continue to promote that paradigm along with research, we can have a growing presence and shift the public into appreciating and utilizing chiropractic care on a regular basis.

What profession other than your own would you like to have attempted?

I really fell in love with chiropractic when I was in my early 20s and honestly I've never looked back. I could be both a yoga and martial arts instructor. I am certified and have all these other skills that I've accumulated and adopted into as much of a wellness lifestyle as I can have. I have pursued different interests but to me it just all enhances my experience with chiropractic.

Are there any other comments you'd like to share about the wonders of chiropractic?

There are two ways I view the profession. I look at it globally and imagine myself as an astronaut or someone taking pictures of the earth, seeing how the sun's rays reflect on the earth from thousands of miles in outer space. I look at the light that comes off the earth and I think to myself, "What degree would the earth be brighter and healthier?"

I couple that with a visual reflection of the earth's population and the increased health and life flowing through their bodies and how the earth would be more illuminated, brighter, more peaceful, whole, and more loving if people were not living in such fear of surgeries, death, and disease the way we are now. If we could examine and adjust the more than six billion people on the planet, we'd have a much healthier population and the planet would work in a much more productive manner.

This is similar to B.J. Palmer's famous words when he wrote about chiropractic and the big picture of the man who slipped on the sidewalk. Small things, like subluxations or adjustments, multiplied by millions, can have huge consequences. He wrote: "The adjustment of the subluxation to release pressure upon nerves, to restore mental impulse flow, to restore health, is big enough to rebuild the thoughts and actions of the world. The idea that knows the cause, that can correct the cause of dis-ease, is one of the biggest ideas known. Without it, nations fall; with it, nations rise. This idea is the biggest I know of."

I love what that says and I really think it's true. I look at it and know that is our role and it is what we are all here to do. We need to find a way to educate and allow people to understand and appreciate the service we offer. We have to collect the data and prove what a positive and spiritual experience it is to receive a chiropractic adjustment, which unites the physical part of a person with the spiritual side, making him or her whole again.

Years from now when people look at your tombstone, what would you want them to read?

I'll tell you a quick story. When we buried my great aunt in Beverly Hills, there was a tombstone about 10 feet from hers and the person who did the voice of Bugs Bunny was laid to rest there. His name was Mel Blanc and on his stone it said, "That's all folks!" Another one I saw read, "I told you I was not feeling well."

Frankly, I don't intend to be buried. I intend to be cremated and have my ashes spread out over the Pacific Ocean somewhere. If anyone remembers me, that's nice, but spiritually speaking I'm just a grain of sand on the beach and just a cog in the wheel and I couldn't care less. I am only concerned about the present and what it is that I'm doing today. Who can I help today? How can I be of service today? And how can I surrender better today?

After his graduation from Logan College of Chiropractic, **Terry A. Rondberg, D.C.,** built successful practices in St. Louis and Phoenix. He was noted for his emphasis on public and patient education and became a staunch advocate of subluxation-based chiropractic.

As publisher of *The Chiropractic Journal* and founder and CEO of the World Chiropractic Alliance, he is a key figure in political lobbying, public education, and intra professional communication. He served on the Department of Defense Chiropractic Advisory Committee to help establish the protocol for making chiropractic services available to active duty military personnel. He also worked closely with global health care officials and organizations, including the World Health Organization.

Dr. Rondberg is also involved in chiropractic research and was instrumental in the formation and administration of the Council on Chiropractic Practice, which developed the profession's only subluxation-centered practice guidelines. In addition, he wrote or co-wrote three books: "Chiropractic First," "Under the Influence of Modern Medicine," and "Chiropractic: Compassion and Expectation."

Armand Rossi

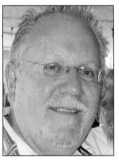

Where are you from originally and what was your childhood like?

I was born in Newark, New Jersey, and raised on the North Jersey Shore, just north of Asbury Park. I really had a good childhood with my parents and sister and family and lively Italian family background. Health-wise, it was not so good until I had chiropractic care around age 5.

What inspired you to get involved with chiropractic?

I was born with asthma and lots of allergies and when I was 5 I fell down a flight of steps. Soon afterwards, I came down with a flu-type sickness that progressed to my being really sick. I couldn't eat and my eyes crossed inward. They took me to a cousin who was a medical doctor on Long Island and he wanted to do surgery right away, to cut the eye muscles and straighten them out. He also wanted to put me in the hospital to see if I had a brain tumor.

Back then, since they didn't have MRIs or CAT scans, they would have had to inject a dye into my skull through my ear and take X-rays. My parents didn't want to go through that — at least not as a first step — so they talked to my mother's uncle, Dr. Frank Fasulo, who was the first chiropractor in my family.

We visited his practice in South Orange, New Jersey, and after checking my spine and nervous system he said I had an Atlas subluxation that could have come from the fall or could have been there from birth. "You can always have the surgery later," he said. "But let's do this first."

My parents agreed that his approach was more conservative and logical so they let him adjust me. He checked me every day but after a few days, when nothing changed, my mother started worrying. My uncle wasn't discouraged though. He pointed out to her that before the adjustment, I had been getting worse every day. Now, at least, I was staying the same, and that was an improvement.

He continued to check my spine and adjust me for the next two or three weeks, and I started eating and feeling more active. One morning, my mother walked into my room and my previously crossed eyes straightened out right in front of her!

I fully recovered from this episode and my mom, typical of people who don't understand chiropractic, was going to have me stop going to my Uncle Frank. "Wait one minute," he lectured her. "He still has nerve interference and his Atlas is still not right, so let's work with that some more."

I started going three times a week, then twice a week, and then once a week. In six months, my allergies started to disappear and by the time I turned 6, my asthma, which the medical doctors said I *might* outgrow by the time I was 12, was completely gone. From then on, going to the doctor meant going to the chiropractor.

> A lot of people get involved in chiropractic because it's a good profession and they can make money and live decently. But they don't necessarily have the passion for chiropractic.

I didn't really think of becoming a chiropractor until the early 1970s. I enrolled at Rutgers University in 1969 and although I never failed a class, my grades weren't very high and in 1971 they kicked me out because my GPA was too low according to their standards.

This was during the Vietnam War and I would have been eligible for the draft unless I was in college. I talked to my Uncle Frank, who convinced me to try chiropractic school. I'm going to be honest with you, at first I did it just to stay out of the draft!

I enrolled at Columbia Institute of Chiropractic in New York City and from the first semester there, I started getting really turned on to chiropractic. My partner in the palpation lab that first quarter, Irene Gold, introduced me to her husband, Reggie Gold, who helped me understand the philosophy of chiropractic. My mother's uncle was a great chiropractor but he never really taught the philosophy the way I learned it from Reggie.

Learning chiropractic became more than simply a way to avoid the draft. I realized I really **wanted** to be a chiropractor! I transferred to Palmer Chiropractic College, where Dr. Gerry Clum was assigned as my student clinician. Gerry and I became very good friends. He was best man at my wedding and we started going to Dynamic Essentials meetings together. Although we may not see each other for months at a time, we're still good friends.

First the Golds and then Gerry. I surely have been blessed to be put in places where I could meet such people.

Where do you currently reside and how are you spending your time these days?

I reside in Boca Raton, Florida, and I have a satellite office there, as well as my main office in Margate, Florida. I see patients four and a half days a week and teach for the International Chiropractic Pediatrics Association (ICPA). Every so often, I'll spend a weekend teaching a module for the ICPA certification program. I've taught and lectured all over the world. This year alone I'll be in Detroit, Chicago, Atlanta, Australia and Canada. In the past, I've been to Amsterdam, Barcelona, Paris, London, Canada, Mexico, and Puerto Rico.

How does the profession differ now from when you first became involved?

When I first became involved, when people entered chiropractic colleges it was kind of a "mission" for them. To enter chiropractic college 33 years ago, you had to be a little off center. You weren't aiming to fit into society and the prevailing paradigm: you wanted to create a new paradigm.

Today, it's a little different because a lot of people get involved in chiropractic because it's a good profession and they can make money and live decently. But they don't necessarily have the passion for chiropractic. Many of us came into chiropractic with the passion, or caught the passion early on. That's what may be lacking a little today. On the other hand, many students are graduating school far better trained to correct subluxations then I was. There is more technology, like surface EMG, and there are better ways to learn. The only problem is, we often over-educate people and they lose sight of the mission.

How do chiropractic and performance relate?

Performance means how you live and how you function. The essence of chiropractic is correcting subluxation to allow you to function — or perform, if you will — at your highest level. It's not a treatment for pain. Although it may help pain, that isn't the goal. The goal is to remove subluxation, to reconnect individuals physically and spiritually, and allow them to perform to their utmost degree.

How does chiropractic relate to a person realizing his or her fullest human potential?

It's like walking into a room where all the lights are on a dimmer switch but they're constantly set for only 75 percent. Most people live their lives that way. Chiropractic makes sure they are living their lives at 100 percent.

That's the essence of chiropractic, which really needs to be taught. You don't need symptoms. You don't need pain. You don't need to be tired and you certainly don't need to be sick. You only need to make sure your life is "turned on" to its fullest potential and you can function at a level you may never have known possible.

How does chiropractic offer people an opportunity to realize an enhanced quality of life?

We find that families that come in together to have their subluxations corrected stay healthier. They enjoy a healthier family environment and there's a bonding that goes on with the family; they do it together like other functions they do together. Lots of times in today's society, people don't get together unless they're at home. Even then, half the time they don't do things together. It works out well for people who experience chiropractic as a family.

What do you feel has happened to the chiropractic profession that may have limited it from being seen by the world in its true nature?

I'll give you two things. One of them is insurance. Insurance deals with treating conditions, so it was easier for chiropractors to buy into the insurance system and treat conditions. But they are not educating people about lifetime care and lifetime potential for being healthier and living a more enhanced life. I won't go so far as to say that by taking health insurance you're selling out, but it's easy for people to make money and then lose sight of the bigger picture. They then have trouble teaching people about it.

The second thing is the over-education in diagnosis and stuff like that. It's made chiropractic more egocentric rather than service-centered. We start thinking that because we learn so much we know so much, when in reality we know very little.

I catch myself at times doing the same thing but I realize I don't know squat about the real things that are going on. Nobody does!

I think it was *Scientific American* that some years ago published an article saying if we compared all the intelligence of the universe to the ocean beaches, "educated" intelligence would be like a single grain of sand on the Atlantic coast.

Now, I want to learn, but understand this: if we doubled all human knowledge, it would be just two grains of sand. Obviously, there's a lot we still don't know. We need to stop thinking we know so much and just go in there, remove interference to the best of our ability, and let the intelligence within each of us take over because **IT** knows what's going on.

I learned from Dr. Sid Williams that any time you get too focused on your own ego — whether it's that you think you're so great, or you find yourself complaining and getting upset or depressed about some meaningless thing — the way to get over it is through pure service. Just serve people and forget about outcomes and attachments to results. Just serve people and you subjugate your ego and connect with the Universal Spirit.

> *Obviously, there's a lot we still don't know. We need to stop thinking we know so much and just go in there, remove interference to the best of our ability, and let the intelligence within each of us take over because IT knows what's going on.*

Chiropractic has become tagged as a pain-relief specialty. In your opinion, what more does it have to offer people?

It should **never** have been a pain relief specialty. Pain relief is almost a side effect of chiropractic. I often tell people that the reconnection of physical and spiritual is what makes you, in the truest sense of the word, holistic — a whole being. Innate Intelligence and the God within you are more fully expressed. Chiropractic takes away the physical barrier that's preventing that Innate force within to be expressed fully throughout your physical being.

What is the purpose of the chiropractic adjustment and how does not receiving chiropractic care impact one's life?

The purpose of the adjustment is to break down any interference between the physical and the spiritual link. Without adjustments, people are not allowing that full expression to exist. There's always some kind of interference there. People can be very spiritual and very in tune but they can only get so far without the adjustment. I believe chiropractic care is totally necessary in order to reach one's fullest spiritual capability in this physical world. My mission is to do my part to make sure everyone on the planet in my lifetime has the opportunity to be checked for subluxation.

What is your favorite quote and how has it impacted your life?

My favorite quote is by B.J. Palmer: "We never know how far reaching something we may think, say or do today will affect the lives of millions tomorrow."

This may sound kind of crazy, but when I first got involved in chiropractic school I was not totally committed to being a chiropractor yet. One night, at a party, I got drunk and I passed out on a friend's couch. I had a dream of this little figure who was like Superman with a cape and he was flying across the sky, although the sky wasn't really the sky — it was the universe.

As he was flying, he was skywriting the words, "We never know how far reaching something we may think, say or do today will affect the lives of millions tomorrow."

I looked at the little character and I saw it was me. I woke up in a solid sweat, which could have been the toxins from the alcohol, I don't know. The fun part of this is that before my dream, I didn't know that quote. I went into the library at Palmer and I asked the lady behind the desk to look at one of B.J. Palmer's *Green Books*.

She asked me which one I wanted and I told her to just pick one. She picked out a book, gave it to me, and I sat down at a table. I opened up the book right in the middle and the first thing I saw was, "We never know how far reaching something we may think, say or do today will affect the lives of millions tomorrow."

When I saw that, I slammed the book shut, gave it back, went home, and lay in bed for the rest of the day. It was then that I realized my life had a bigger purpose.

How is chiropractic unique and what does it offer that other health professions do not?

We are the only profession that purposefully corrects interference, the subluxation. No other profession does that deliberately. Now, a person can go to an osteopath and get manipulated and it may correct interference. But it was not done intentionally for that. That's what makes chiropractic totally unique.

What do you sense was the intention behind the creation of chiropractic?

If we're talking about D.D. Palmer and Harvey Lillard, I think it was the first *intentional* act of putting together the cause and effect relationship of the neurological system. Chiropractic was born when we began to understand how interference was involved with the neurological system.

In the very beginning, they thought the subluxation was the cause of all disease. I think the focus of the profession has evolved to be the correction of interference, which allows the physical and spiritual to reconnect. It isn't a treatment for disease even though, in the beginning — through the latter part of D.D. Palmer's life and the early involvement of his son, B.J. Palmer — it was considered more of a treatment of all disease.

I think the focus of the profession has evolved to be the correction of interference, which allows the physical and spiritual to reconnect. It isn't a treatment for disease even though, in the beginning... it was considered more of a treatment of all disease.

Who are some of your mentors and what impact have they had on your life?

The first would be my mother's uncle, because of what he did when I was so sick. The next one would be Reggie Gold, because I learned philosophy through him. The next two would probably be Sid Williams and Gerry Clum, by watching what they have done in and for the profession.

Another one was Joe Flesia from the chiropractic Renaissance movement. I was very blessed to have had many private talks with Joe when he was creating Renaissance with Guy Riekeman. Joe certainly helped me a lot.

Then after that it would be Dr. Albert Reach, from whom I learned much about how to achieve a high volume in my office. He taught me how to break down some of the barriers within myself. Al Reach's mentor, Dr. James Sigafoose, became my mentor as well. When I learned everything I could learn from Al, I looked to see who taught him and learned that it was Dr. Sigafoose. So, I became friends with him and we're pretty close even now.

What are some things, if any, you had to give up in order to devote your life to chiropractic?

I've had to give up some of my attachments to money, prestige, and things like that to really devote my life to chiropractic. I remember in the early days of school — and this may sound kind of silly — I used to play guitar and I had to give that up because the calluses on my fingers made it hard to feel things. You know, I don't feel that I've given up as much as I've received.

What turns you on creatively, spiritually, or emotionally?

A good movie and walking out by the ocean. I love listening to people who tell me what chiropractic has done for them, whether they're my patients or someone else's. I love listening to that. Even though there are so many more people we never hear from, it's a blessing to get that kind of feedback.

One of the neatest things is when I'm teaching a seminar and I see students' eyes light up. It's an "ah ha" moment for them — they get it! Traveling and doing the seminars can be tiring sometimes but when I see that, feel that, or hear that, or when someone writes to me that I made a difference, that's neat.

> **I see the profession split. I think part of chiropractic will split off into a different type of profession. They'll be called doctors of alternative medicine and use manipulation as a form of treatment of disease, the same as they would use nutrition, massage, acupuncture, etc.**

Where do you see the profession 10 years from now?

I see the profession split. I think part of chiropractic will split off into a different type of profession. They'll be called doctors of alternative medicine and use manipulation as a form of treatment of disease, the same as they would use nutrition, massage, acupuncture, etc.

The others will remain principled chiropractors working with the subluxation. I don't see this split as a bad thing necessarily, because there will be a place for people who are doctors of alternative medicine and the two don't have to be in conflict.

What profession other than your own would you like to have attempted?

My goodness, I don't know. Musician maybe. I find that music and chiropractic work hand-in-hand because of the art. There's a philosophy, science, and art in each. When you're a musician, the art is very similar to the art of chiropractic. In chiropractic, I see chiropractors who are adjusting people strictly by procedure and that's like a musician playing an instrument by notes. It isn't music or the true artistic expression of music, any more than adjusting people by procedure is the true artistic expression of chiropractic.

The true way to express these two similar arts is through emotion. In music, it's by feeling what the composer was trying to portray with the music. In chiropractic, you feel the person, the tone, and the energy. You understand the science behind what you're doing, but you feel and sense what needs to be done.

As far as the tone is concerned, Drs. Gentempo and Kent did a study that showed tissue cells become denser in a subluxated area. I have found, by palpation, areas of relative density that are associated with areas of subluxation. That's part of the sense of feeling — what I call relative density — which is part of the art.

What got you involved with the pediatric aspect of chiropractic?

That was kind of interesting. When I moved from Phoenix to Atlanta, I hooked up with Dr. Larry Webster. I had met Larry years before and he had even shown me the Webster Breech Turning Technique. Larry, along with Eddie Cohen, asked me if I wanted to teach in their ICPA certification program, which was just getting started.

My response was, "Larry, I'm not a pediatric expert." He had people like Claudia Anrig, Judy Forrester, Palmer and Jennifer Peet, Joe Flesia, and other people I considered *real* pediatric experts. Larry said to me, "When you had your big practice in Arizona, how many people did you see?" I told him 900 to 1,000 patient visits a week. He asked, "How many were kids?" I thought about it, and answered, "A good 30 percent." That's about 300 patient visits a week for kids alone. He said, "Do you realize that you are seeing more kids than the experts are?" I told him I didn't think of it that way, but that's the reason he wanted me on the program.

Are there any other comments you have about the wonders of chiropractic that you would like to share?

Simply that it changes lives, changes people, changes society, and that we are just scratching the surface right now. I think the biggest thing is to never put a limit on chiropractic. Never tell people that chiropractic can't help them if they have cancer or whatever else it may be. One of the best lines Al Reach taught me was, "If you are alive and have nerve interference, don't you think you would be better off **without** the interference whether you have symptoms or not?"

Years from now when people look at your tombstone, what would you want them to read?

"He was a guy who cared." That's it.

Armand M. Rossi, D.C., a 1976 graduate of Palmer College of Chiropractic, currently practices in Margate and Boca Raton, Florida. Formerly the instructor of Pediatric Adjusting at Life University, Dr. Rossi practiced in Smyrna, Georgia from 1977 to 1982 and then moved to Phoenix where he practiced and supervised one of the largest chiropractic office groups in the world until returning to Georgia in 1993.

Dr. Rossi is a "Fellow" and a teaching member of the International Chiropractic Pediatric Association, and holds membership in the International Chiropractors Association. He also belongs to the Florida Chiropractic Society, which in 2008 presented him with its "Chiropractor of the Year" award.

A lecturer who travels the world teaching other chiropractors about pediatric chiropractic, Dr. Rossi considers having two and three generations of chiropractic patients receive care on a regular basis as his most prestigious honor. He and his wife, Terry, live in Boca Raton and have four children, nine grandchildren, and two great-grandchildren.

James Sigafoose

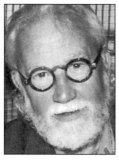

Who inspired you to get involved with chiropractic?

My father.

Where are you from originally and what was your childhood like?

I'm from Baltimore. I had a good childhood.

Where do you currently reside and how are you spending your time these days?

I work. If you call what I do work. I do not call it work. I travel around the world doing seminars and I live right outside of Baltimore. I teach philosophy in my seminars. I talk about chiropractic, which is not being taught in schools, so I teach it.

How does the profession of chiropractic differ now from when you first became involved?

Well, it was more chiropractic-based and the Palmers taught *chiropractic* at that time, which they don't do anymore. It was more chiropractic than it was therapy. Today, I think it's closer to the practice of medicine than ever.

How do chiropractic and performance relate?

Chiropractic is a way of life and the end purpose is to correct subluxations to allow a greater infusion of Innate Intelligence through matter, period. Everybody is better off by being adjusted. Yet, there are people who live to be 105 or 110 who never had an adjustment so I can't say that chiropractic enhances performance. What I *can* say is that everybody is better off by being adjusted.

What do you feel chiropractic has to offer to people who get adjustments versus those who do not?

Well, they at least have a rise in potential. They have an opportunity to have a potential that is greater than they have at present, mentally, physically, and spiritually. That is the extent of that.

How does chiropractic relate to a person realizing his or her fullest human potential?

If the corrective adjustment is made (which is not always done) at the right place (which is not always done) the individual has the opportunity to function physically, mentally, and spiritually at a higher potential. The adjustments are not just racking up 206 bones. The adjustment is unlocking a specific bone in the spine and allowing Innate to set it where it belongs because only Innate knows where it belongs — no one else does.

What is Innate?

Innate, to me, is God.

What do you feel has happened to chiropractic that may have limited it from being seen by the world in its true nature?

Education. What do they educate you about? They educate you about everything **but** chiropractic. At one time, chiropractic was primarily about the spinal anatomy, the philosophy, the principle of chiropractic, and how to relate that. I don't think they teach that anymore. As a matter of fact, I *know* they don't. They have, at some of the schools, eliminated subluxation. They have eliminated the teaching of Innate. They have eliminated that which is chiropractic so what you have is a therapy.

What do you feel we need to do as a profession, if anything, to get the profession back on track?

Introduce the basics of chiropractic and the fundamentals of chiropractic into the teaching rather than attempt to make chiropractors great diagnosticians and great therapists and great pseudo-medical doctors. Make them great chiropractors.

Chiropractic has become tagged as a pain relief specialty. In your opinion what more does chiropractic have to offer people?

I do not think that chiropractic has anything to do with pain. Chiropractic doesn't treat symptoms, it doesn't treat diseases, it doesn't treat anything. That is a misnomer completely. Chiropractic is the ability to correct the subluxation. The ability to find the subluxation is the analysis, and once the analysis has been made and the correction has been made, then Innate does its work.

In all of your years in chiropractic, what have you seen and how have you witnessed Innate doing its work?

If you're talking about the effect of Innate, anything from healing blind eyes to deaf ears, cancers to crippling conditions to drug addiction. Add to that changes in spiritual being, increased mental faculties, even changes of dietary intake.

At one time, we took care of tons of people in Yoga ashrams. These street people were on dope and weren't very hygienic and eventually, over a period of time, without a spoken word, they got off these drugs, began to clean themselves up, and even dress better without anyone speaking to them about it. It's something I suppose they realized was necessary once they became more functional.

I've never really considered chiropractic a health profession. What chiropractic does for the world at large is simply allow a greater expression of Innate through matter.

What is the purpose of the chiropractic adjustment and how does not receiving chiropractic impact one's life?

Well, that's a simple thing! The purpose is to allow maximum expression of Innate through matter. Without it, matter is incapable of functioning the way it was designed. Not receiving chiropractic adjustments prevents the expression of Innate from occurring at its maximum potential.

What is your favorite quote and how has it impacted your life?

My favorite quote? I don't know that I have one.

How is chiropractic unique and what does it offer that other health professions do not?

Well, I'm just not certain. I've never really considered chiropractic a health profession. What chiropractic does for the world at large is simply allow a greater expression of Innate through matter. Universal Intelligence and Innate Intelligence are the same thing. Innate Intelligence is within all living entities and Universal Intelligence is in everything. Universal Intelligence can be destructive whereas Innate Intelligence is never destructive. For instance, we have lightning, floods, earthquakes, tornadoes, hurricanes, and these are all things done to maintain a balance in the universe, which is behind Universal Intelligence and Universal Law.

What do you sense was the intention behind the creation of chiropractic?

I think that chiropractic always existed. I couldn't tell you when it was created; I would say it is part of life itself. When it was recognized as a profession in 1895, it was more or less by accident. When giving an adjustment, they found that certain things occurred that shifted the body from dysfunction to function.

Then they applied the principles of chiropractic to the teaching of a particular profession. At one time, it was going to be a religion and they decided against making it a religion and made it a profession that was available to everybody who wanted it.

I think chiropractic today would be better off, for many reasons, if it had originally become a religion. For one thing, it may not have shifted over into physical medicine. Also, we would be tax free and that would be a wonderful thing! Freedom is another reason it would have been better as a religion. Not being dictated to by governments, the so-called state boards, and the reach of controlling factors that have nothing to do with chiropractic.

Do you feel it's too late for the profession to get back on track and be seen by the world in its true nature?

As it is now, schools are producing high-quality and highly educated ambitious doctors, but without the message. They have no understanding what chiropractic is, nor the ability to teach it, preach it, or to offer it even. The concept of chiropractic being taught is no more than physical medicine, period.

Salvation for us requires two things. Number one, we need to have Innate Consciousness Centers throughout the United States and the world. We already have one in the making in Fort Myers, Florida.

The second thing is to have a public relations program by a real public relations company. In fact, we already have a PR outfit — the same PR outfit that works for Merck, Pfizer, and all the large drug companies. They have agreed to take chiropractic on as a client and have already built a website for us. What we need now is a minimum of a thousand chiropractors who will get off their wallet and contribute about $45 a week for the enhancement of chiropractic through the web. The message would go worldwide and certainly increase the level of education of the people on planet earth as to what chiropractic actually is. The website is at chirousa.com and chiropractors can go online and contribute to this great cause.

Who are some of your mentors and what impact have they had on your life?

Clark Rich of Clearfield, Pennsylvania, was my mentor who helped me immensely in my transformation from being a pseudo-medical doctor to a chiropractor. The others were Sid Williams, B.J. Palmer, and Jesus Christ — in that order. I think it's self evident about their mentorship.

Clark Rich was a highly principled chiropractor whose life was chiropractic. He was a tremendous giver of information, love, and all the things that are necessary for a mentor. He was great. Of course, Sid Williams has always been a die-hard chiropractor whose whole being is to teach and preach principled chiropractic. And we all know about Jesus! Well, at least we **should** know, and that's self-evident.

What are some things that you have had to give up, if any, in order to devote your life to chiropractic?

I don't know that I had to give anything up, to tell you the truth. First of all, I didn't know I had some of the gifts I had; I had to learn that. Toastmasters International helped me recognize that I had ability for public speaking. That was a great revelation for me and I didn't have to give anything up there. Maybe if I gave anything up at all it was more closeness with my family. When I became highly dedicated to having the practice I had — which was 2,000 visits a week — I may have neglected some of the things I could have done and should have done with my family. We always traveled together. I'd take them on trips around the world and I took them to all the seminars that I went to. They weren't neglected by any means. It's just that perhaps I wasn't as attentive to them as I could have been. That probably is the greatest sacrifice I've made.

What turns you on creatively, spiritually, or emotionally?

I don't know that anything "turns me on." It's either there or it isn't. I think that my greatest love is speaking and giving seminars. When I do a seminar, things come to me that I hadn't really thought about or didn't even think I knew about. So, that's a form of creation. I would say doing seminars is the biggest one and involves all of those things above.

Where do you see the profession 10 years from now?

If it continues the way it is, it will be no different than osteopathy was a few years ago. Osteopathy was once a separate and distinct science, art, and philosophy, but now it's really no different than the practice of medicine. Within a 10-year period, the word chiropractic will exist, but the practice and the philosophy and so on won't — unless we do something drastically different than we are doing now.

The only thing that can save chiropractic as I know it is the profession. If only 1,000 chiropractors dedicated themselves to the support of this public relations program we have created, that would make a big impact! It's already built and one man has invested almost half a million dollars in it. He's not even a chiropractor, but he feels the need for people to understand chiropractic and get away from drugs and those kinds of things. So, here we have someone who's not even in our own profession doing this for us and we still don't have the profession backing it the way they should. It's my belief that if we embrace this, we could and would save real chiropractic because the public would demand it from chiropractors.

> **Within a 10-year period, the word chiropractic will exist, but the practice and the philosophy and so on won't — unless we do something drastically different than we are doing now.**

The other thing is, we have a lot of people out there in chiropractic who call themselves "gurus" who teach people how to suck more money out of insurance companies and how to make more money. It's all about business and procedure but very little, if anything, about principled chiropractic

We need more people teaching and living the chiropractic life. Christianity is not a religion. Christianity is a philosophy and a way of living. Chiropractic is not a job or a workplace; it's a way of living. If you embrace the way of living and you embrace the principles of chiropractic, you become directly and absolutely different from the way the world thinks. The Bible says that when you become a Christian, you become *peculiar to the world* because you don't think and act like the world. If you become a chiropractor and you really understand the philosophy and the principle of chiropractic, you become very peculiar to other professions, so-called health professions. As a matter of fact, you become very peculiar to your fellow chiropractors for the most part.

Do you want to share more about the creation of these Innate Consciousness Centers?

When chiropractors have patients who are not responding to whatever they're doing, they can send them to these places. Again, the first one we have is in Fort Myers, Florida. They would go to this center where they would be adjusted and taught about Innate. They would be taught about diet. Children would come in and be shown how to eat properly. We would teach people how to cook properly. There would be dancing and massages. Not that those are part of chiropractic, but we are talking about a consciousness of life, understanding life, and the practice of living the Innate way.

The Innate way is to get away from drugs, to do things to the body that will enhance the function of the body, and particularly be adjusted specifically. People going to the center would be checked for subluxations regularly. They would spend a week, two weeks, three weeks, a month, or whatever time they needed to learn how to change their life. They would leave there in a month's time — or even a week's time — with a whole new idea of how they should treat their body.

What are some things that are being practiced in the chiropractor's office that in your mind does not have a place there?

Therapy.

What are the things chiropractors should be doing in their offices?

Teaching chiropractic and adjusting people specifically. What is the purpose of adjusting and doing all of this stuff to extremities in all the bones all over the body? And they say, "That's what D.D. taught."

Let's realize we have a brain. We have a brain that enters through the foramen magnum, that enters into the first two bones in the neck and goes down through the spinal column. The health of the spinal column is essential to the health of the physical being. Since there is a direct relationship between the physical being and the mental being, and a direct relationship between the mental being and the spiritual being, if we were to have a healthy spine that was maintained healthfully throughout life, we would have a higher potential of life mentally, physically, and spiritually.

B.J. Palmer talked several times about how prostitutes came in and got adjusted and afterwards, they were no longer prostitutes. They simply changed; they could see the difference. Criminals can change and people as a whole can change from being a lower form of life to a higher form of life by having a greater expression of Innate through matter.

It's a hell of a gift from God to man and one that man can give to other people. But it's simply totally and completely misunderstood and misrepresented. Instead, we have these so-called pain clinics and the damn stretchomatics (decompression tables). You're supposed to put somebody on a stretching machine?

It seems that many chiropractors are treating their patients or looking to cure them of something and most are disappointed. What is occurring there?

That's what I'm telling you — that's what they teach. I was at a school in Melbourne, Australia, and their philosophy teacher said the school's mission was to make its students the greatest diagnosticians in the world.

What's diagnosis got to do with chiropractic? It doesn't have anything to do with it. What do they teach the students in school? If the symptoms aren't gone they need to go to therapy. What was once a great chiropractic school is now giving IV hydration to a rugby team. That chiropractic college was once a very straight chiropractic school and now they're giving IVs for dehydration? Now you tell me if that's chiropractic.

What profession other than your own would you like to have attempted?

At one time, I thought in terms of veterinary medicine, but that isn't where I was led. My father painted a picture of me being a chiropractor since I was about 4 years old.

Are there any other comments you'd like to share about the wonders of chiropractic?

It's not how broad the stroke of the brush is, it's how fine it is and how thinly lined and specific it is. It's not how much you do to a person, it's what you do to them. The less you do, the better. The concept out there now is to move every bone in the body, manipulate every joint that exists in the body, heat 'em, cool 'em, stretch 'em, and do everything possible to invade the body in some manner rather than just one simple thing: locate one bone that is out of alignment, correct it, be sure it is corrected, maintain its correction, and give it time (which is the sixth principle in chiropractic) to resurrect the body as a whole from a subatomic particle to a solid mass.

What better gift is there to give somebody than the opportunity to receive maximum expression of life? What good is your body without life? You can't add life to it, but you most certainly can increase the expression of life to all the tissue cells, thus giving normal function, normal vibration, and normal action of the cell from a subatomic particle to the total organism. What's better than that? What's greater than that?

And what do drugs do? Drugs don't do that! Drugs do one of two things. They either inhibit or stimulate the function of the body or they attempt to destroy a negative cell. At the same time, they reduce the immune system and destroy a lot of healthy tissues. You don't gain health from taking drugs.

When you have a major subluxation, you lose life and you gain death. When you correct that subluxation and maintain that correction long enough, which is the only time the body does any healing, you, in fact, are losing death and gaining life.

We need centers that can teach large numbers of people, particularly people who were dying or on their way out, how to prepare food and get them to ask themselves questions like: "What foods should I be eating?" (Raw, high-energy foods, of course!) ... "What is the chiropractic adjustment?" ... "How does it work?" ... "Why does it work?" ... "What is its purpose?" ... "What is Innate?" ... "What is life itself?" ... "What is God?" ... "Who is God?" ... "Where is God?" ... "What kind of relationship do I have with God?"

You can boil it all down to this: When your physical body separates or is separated to any degree from God, it begins to dysfunction and die. When you have a major subluxation, you lose life and you gain death. When you correct that subluxation and maintain that correction long enough, which is the only time the body does any healing, you, in fact, are losing death and gaining life.

That's a pretty wonderful gift I would think we give to people. But here in the United States of America, we have the Constitution, which is common law and common law is God's law. When we started to change the Constitution, we began to separate the nation from God. The violation of the Constitution is a major subluxation that affects the function of our country and the subluxation is a violation of the principle or the law that runs us, which is called the law of life.

As we separate ourselves from God, we become diseased.

You know, people don't agree with everything I say, but I don't really care whether they agree with me or not. I see the parallel between chiropractic and our country. If we would go back to the basic fundamentals that created and made this country wonderful and great, we would have a healthy country today.

The same goes for chiropractic. Some of our best chiropractors knew only about the spine and the philosophy — that's all they knew and that's all they practiced. They did very well and they thrived. Today, people who practice real chiropractic, who continue to teach chiropractic and live chiropractic, no matter what the so-called economic situation is, are going to survive and thrive.

If people are really concerned about other people and about the welfare of this world, they should learn what chiropractic is. Not what they were taught at school... but what chiropractic truly is as it was taught by the founders of chiropractic...

You've been wonderful, as always, and I appreciate your time. Is there anything else you would like to share?

If people are really concerned about other people and about the welfare of this world, they should learn what chiropractic is. Not what they were taught at school or what the common person has been led to believe, but what chiropractic truly is as it was taught by the founders of chiropractic and the researchers of chiropractic, true researchers, not just B.J. Palmer.

Every chiropractor on earth should be reading all of the *Green Books*. Some say that's antiquated chiropractic and it doesn't exist anymore. Bull crap! Gravity still exists and all of the universal laws still exist. Chiropractic very definitely falls under the category of universal law.

If students and the public were taught these things by people who researched these principles and gave their lives to them, they would, through modeling, change their own thinking and lives.

We do a seminar program called The Gathering where the whole purpose is to change people's thinking. Once you change your thinking, you change your environment through action. It does no good just to think about it ... you have to have the thought and then be able to act upon it before you can get any result.

The whole purpose of a Gathering (and I'm not promoting the

seminars, I'm just promoting the idea) is to help you get rid of your fears, hang-ups, and blocks so you can be more clear about who you are, what you are, and what you are dealing with, which is chiropractic!

We have another program called The Systems, which is a mentoring program, not a coaching program. If you're able to receive a constant flow of information that is moving you gently (and sometimes not so gently) toward being a very fundamental, principled chiropractic office, you are going to be successful. You can't fight success when you maintain the fundamentals and the principles of chiropractic. It's a natural.

Years from now when people look at your tombstone, what would you want them to read?

We'll meet again some sunny day.

In 1968, after having failed in chiropractic for seven years, **James Sigafoose, D.C.,** attended Dr. Sid Williams' Dynamic Essentials (DE) seminar. There he learned philosophy and went on to build the largest volume chiropractic office in the world during the 1970s. He is now recognized worldwide for his inspirational chiropractic philosophy and motivational skills, especially as a team teacher with Parker Seminars for 15 years and DE for more than 45 years.

Dr. Sigafoose has spoken internationally in countries such as Japan and Australia in 1989 and 1990, and has been honored as "Chiropractor of the Year" many times. For more than 25 years, he has helped doctors overcome their fears and be better chiropractors through his "Gatherings" seminars.

He has written many books and presented a variety of audio and video offerings, which serve as educational materials for chiropractors all over the world. Dr. Sigafoose married Patsy in 1954 and all six surviving children became chiropractors — as well as a son-in-law, nephew, and daughter-in-law.

You must live in the present, launch yourself on every wave, find your eternity in each moment. Fools stand on their island of opportunities and look toward another land. There is no other land; there is no other life but this.

Henry David Thoreau

Joe Strauss

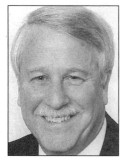

Where are you from originally and what was your childhood like?

I was born in Philadelphia and we moved to the suburbs in 1952. A man named William Levitt built 17,000 homes in Bucks County, Pennsylvania, and my family moved there when I was 7 years old. I grew up there and I had a great childhood. My father had his own ice cream stand business, so you know it had to be a great childhood! I worked in that business from the time I was 13, from washing dishes to working the counter making ice cream cones and sundaes.

I knew by the time I was 15 that I wanted to be a chiropractor. My uncle was a chiropractor and I thought that it was just really an interesting profession. I took the credits I needed in college in order to get licensed in Pennsylvania. I think it was just six credits each in physics, chemistry, and biology. I lived at home and worked at my dad's ice cream store until I went off to chiropractic college.

What inspired you to get involved with chiropractic?

I had thought about going into dentistry, but I knew chiropractic was a clean profession and there was no blood involved. I really didn't know a whole lot about chiropractic until I injured my back wrestling in high school. My mother was actually the first one to go to my uncle. He went to school for chiropractic and opened his practice late in life. My mom had a real bad case of tendonitis, partially from working at the store. We used to sell frozen mugs of root beer and she'd carry four to five at a time and ended up with an inflamed elbow. During the time she was going to my uncle, I had my injury and it was so bad I couldn't even swing a baseball bat. I went to the chiropractor and, as a side effect

231

of the adjustments, my summer allergies cleared up as well. That was a positive experience with chiropractic and it seemed like a good profession.

Where do you currently reside and how are you spending your time these days?

I never really left Levittown. After school (I went to the Columbia Institute of Chiropractic in Manhattan) my wife and I moved back home right next to my parent's house, which my sister had bought as an investment property. We opened our first office there.

After living there for four and a half years, we decided we needed more room because the practice was growing considerably and we wanted more space. Plus, kids were on the way. A vacant lot was for sale on the other side of town. We wanted to build a home-office combination because that's how we started out and we really liked that idea. The lot wasn't quite big enough but it was zoned professional.

We kind of forgot about it and, three months later, we saw an advertisement for a house for sale in a professionally zoned area. I talked to my real estate agent and he told me where it was. To our amazement, the house for sale was right behind the vacant lot we had considered!

We bought the house and vacant lot as two separate properties. We moved into the house in September 1971 and broke ground for the office the day after Thanksgiving of '71 and by February of '72, we were in the new building. We have been there ever since and I have a 40-foot walk to work in the morning between these two separate properties. It has been a great place to live. The house is on a little side street, but the office faces a main street and is a good location.

These days I am in kind of a part-time practice in that I "only" work 40 hours a week! I work Monday, Wednesday, and Friday from nine in the morning until nine at night. I work those three 12 hour days and I still work Saturday morning for four hours. On Tuesdays and Thursdays, I try to do some writing. I write a lot of books and publish a chiropractic philosophy newsletter called "The Pivot Review."

I write a practice-building newsletter as well as educational materials. Today, I'm working on a presentation for the Garden State Chiropractic Society. I also play on a senior softball team and we play 40 games from April through October. Once in a while, I get out and ride my motorcycle. I am also into exercising and go to the gym Tuesday, Thursday, and one weekend day. I travel and speak on chiropractic. I have been to Japan twice, once to New Zealand, England, Canada, and various engagements throughout the United States.

How does the profession differ now from when you first became involved?

The big difference is that when I first went into practice, people were not very familiar with what chiropractic was all about and you really had a good opportunity to educate them.

Now, people are familiar with chiropractic but, unfortunately, they're usually wrong! The big challenge we have today is changing the perspective of people who have a preconceived idea that chiropractic is about bad backs and stiff necks.

You have to explain to them that it's not about the back; it's about life and expressing full potential and allowing the Innate Intelligence of the body to function without interference in the nerve system due to vertebral subluxation.

That's harder today because most patients think they know what chiropractic is since they've seen the ads in the Yellow Pages or heard about it from other chiropractors. They just assume that if you're going to a chiropractor, it's because you have a bad back, a stiff neck, or some other musculoskeletal problem.

Most patients think they know what chiropractic is since they've seen the ads in the Yellow Pages or heard about it from other chiropractors. They just assume that if you're going to a chiropractor, it's because you have a bad back, a stiff neck, or some other musculoskeletal problem.

How do chiropractic and performance relate?

Performance is clearly one aspect of what chiropractic does but the profession has not really emphasized that aspect. It's been only recently that people like Reggie Gold and others have stressed the idea that performance is important.

But performance is only one aspect of chiropractic. Another is maintaining health, enabling the body to have greater ability to heal itself. I'm sure that's of interest to people who are sick and walk into a chiropractor's office. They need to understand that we aren't going to treat their condition or illness but we are going to make sure that the Innate Intelligence is expressing itself so that their body can have a greater capacity to heal itself.

Performance, health maintenance, and proper function within the body are all ramifications of chiropractic. Performance is an important issue, whether it's athletic performance, academics, housework, your golf game, job efficiency, or other areas.

How does chiropractic relate to a person realizing his or her fullest human potential?

Having a good nerve supply will obviously allow you to reach your fullest human potential. Of course, human potential means different things to different people. We may need to quantify what human potential really is: performance, longevity, enjoyment, and happiness? Obviously, chiropractic touches upon everything that the Innate Intelligence of the body is involved with and everything that the nerve system is involved with, which is just about everything.

How does chiropractic offer people an opportunity to realize an enhanced quality of life?

Every aspect of your life is dependent upon the function of your nerve system. Correcting subluxation is going to enhance your immune system, your nerve system function, your ability to get well if you have physical ailments, your ability to stay well, and even your thinking capacity.

One of the important areas we don't often consider is how understanding the chiropractic philosophy of life — or the Above-Down, Inside-Out philosophy — can enhance life because it gives you a greater perspective on life. It provides an opportunity to realize we have to take responsibility for our own life, whether it's our health, finances, or social life. The "ADIO" philosophy gets people to look at causes rather than effects.

What do you feel has happened to the chiropractic profession that may have limited it from being seen by the world in its true nature?

A lot of factors have caused that. People entering the profession now have not been exposed to chiropractic like I was. I didn't understand the philosophy until I sat my first week of school when this chiropractor from Spring Valley, New York — Dr. Reggie Gold — started to explain what chiropractic was.

My uncle never explained these things to me, although I still had a positive experience with chiropractic. When Reggie started teaching the philosophy, my eyes just opened and things started to click about what we had here in chiropractic.

When they're in school today, students aren't being taught philosophy, so they're not even exposed to the concept of Innate Intelligence. On many chiropractic campuses, that's a term of derision! That drifting away from the philosophy is a factor.

When you drift from the philosophy you drift into the medical model, and trying to squeeze chiropractic into the medical model is moving us completely away from the thing that makes us unique and distinct.

We deal with the Innate Intelligence of the body and its fullest expression. When you get away from that, you get into the therapeutic or medical model. That's definitely a factor that influenced the state of chiropractic today.

When you drift from the philosophy you drift into the medical model, and trying to squeeze chiropractic into the medical model is moving us completely away from the thing that makes us unique and distinct.

The insurance industry and the therapeutic model it embraces have also moved us away from our uniqueness and truth. That's really sad because we've graduated many thousands of new chiropractors, yet there's no way they can be successful in the medical model since they're competing with all other therapeutic practitioners.

We've lost the niche we had (if we ever really had it to begin with) of chiropractic being about life and maintaining the fullest expression of the Innate Intelligence.

Chiropractic has become tagged as a pain relief specialty. In your opinion, what more does it have to offer people?

What it has to offer is the full expression of the Innate Intelligence of your body, which affects every aspect of life.

People need to understand that chiropractic care is about a life-enhancing experience and, unfortunately, we don't explain that clearly enough. We don't explain the full idea of how fantastic the body is, with its ability to heal itself, run itself, and maintain itself in a state of well-being.

Some people emphasize performance, which is better than just treating bad backs and stiff necks. But there's so much more to chiropractic than just performance. Your body is going to last longer if you're under chiropractic care. It's going to have greater ability to heal itself and normalize itself when and if you get sick. All of that is encompassed by the idea of the Innate Intelligence of the body expressing itself more fully when you are subluxation-free.

That's where our emphasis needs to be. Unfortunately most chiropractors don't talk about Innate Intelligence in their office and 90 percent of them probably never even heard the term! Part of the problem is that people just don't understand this whole idea of how fantastic the body is and how chiropractic care relates to every aspect of their lives.

What is the purpose of the chiropractic adjustment and how does not receiving chiropractic care impact one's life?

Part of the problem is that people just don't understand this whole idea of how fantastic the body is and how chiropractic care relates to every aspect of their lives.

The purpose of the chiropractic adjustment is to allow the Innate Intelligence of the body to express itself more fully. Innate Intelligence is a principle of life that is placed within every living organism for the purpose of carrying on life: adapting, assimilating, growing, and reproducing. Innate Intelligence is the principle B.J. Palmer called the "Law of Life," that resides within every living organism whether human beings, plants, or other animals.

Its function is to aid in every aspect of the human experience. In human beings, that principle expresses itself, among other ways, through the nerve system and the vertebral subluxation interferes with that expression. Not receiving chiropractic adjustments impedes the body's ability to work as it should to its fullest potential.

What is your favorite quote and how has it impacted your life?

Giving group lay lectures once a week was a key to the success of my practice. I had a downstairs meeting room that held 40-50 people and on the heating duct in the center of the room was a sign with the B.J. Palmer quote, "You never know how far reaching something you think, say or do today will affect the lives of millions tomorrow."

Every night when I walked down the steps to do that talk, whether there were two people in the room or 20, I would look at that quote and realize what I had to say was important, life changing, and life enhancing.

Those two people would be affected and they would affect hundreds and thousands of others in their lifetime. It made me realize that my talk was important to the growth of my practice and to however many people were there. The saying affected my enthusiasm and desire to make the philosophy clear and applicable to their lives.

What do you sense was the intention behind the creation of chiropractic?

D.D. Palmer and B.J. Palmer realized there was a non-material aspect of human beings that was important and vital to health and life, and that no profession in the world was addressing that immaterial part or how it affected the material part.

Doctors were addressing the material part of the human being, and theologians, clergy, and some of the Christian Science people were trying to address the immaterial part of man — whether they saw it as the soul, spirit, or some other thing. No one addressed the union of the immaterial, the Innate Intelligence, and the physical matter of the body. They stumbled across a means by which the immaterial relates to, addresses, and expresses itself through the material. I think that is what they were trying to do.

Who are some of your mentors and what impact have they had on your life?

Reggie Gold was my greatest mentor from a chiropractic standpoint. I had the privilege of hearing him and over the years becoming friends with him and sharing chiropractic with him. Early in practice, Jim Sigafoose helped quite a bit when I decided to start doing lay lectures. He generated in me much of the enthusiasm I have for chiropractic because he was a dynamic and enthusiastic person. I got much of that from him.

Joe Donofrio has probably been my oldest friend in chiropractic. We went to school together and were in the same class. I taught for 15 years in chiropractic school and many students were my mentors, not necessarily because they taught me anything (although they did on occasion) but because they questioned and challenged my thinking, caused me to investigate, and think further about chiropractic.

I enjoy listening to and reading David Koch; he challenges my thinking as well.

Certainly Thom Gelardi has been another person who over the years has influenced me. Then there have been my friends in chiropractic who I just bounced chiropractic off of over the years — and they bounced things off of me! I try to learn from everybody, even people I might not agree with. The Palmers and their writings have mentored me, challenged my thinking, and made me draw my philosophy to a finer point.

What turns you on creatively, spiritually, or emotionally?

Creatively, finding ways of expressing chiropractic more clearly, ways in which I can relate chiropractic to the average person, challenge their thinking and make them begin to think from an Above-Down, Inside-Out viewpoint.

I try to make chiropractic as understandable as possible because I think sometimes we tend to complicate it. Trying to make chiropractic as simple and understandable as possible is where I focus my creativity.

Spiritually, I am a Born-Again Christian, so my relationship with God and my Lord Jesus Christ is where I get my spiritual thinking and emphasis. Most of my family members are either chiropractors or ministers so at family gatherings we get together over spiritual and chiropractic things. That's an important aspect of my spiritual life, along with reading and studying the Bible. I've actually gone to the University and taken a couple of semesters of Greek in order to be able to understand it better. That has been a part of my spiritual growth.

Emotionally, it's my role as a servant to humanity. Knowing I offer a service that everybody in the world needs — and everybody in the world should have available to them — gets me ramped up emotionally. I have an opportunity and a privilege to serve people through chiropractic. That's important to me emotionally, although I sometimes have to restrain my emotions around people who aren't receptive to chiropractic. I have to recognize intellectually and mentally what I'm doing, which is promoting an understanding of the chiropractic philosophy to everybody I come in contact with. Having somebody new walk into the office really charges me up because I can expose someone to something he or she has never heard before, at least not in this way. That's an exciting thing and gets me revved up.

Where do you see the profession 10 years from now?

That depends on where the profession sees itself. If the profession sees itself as providing a separate, unique, and distinct service to humanity that allows the Innate Intelligence of the body to express itself by correction of the vertebral subluxation, we'll go in the direction I'd like to see us go and we'll succeed as a profession.

If we go the other way and choose the medical model, the way many in our profession are already doing, we'll go the same way osteopathy has gone. We will be smaller in number, non-existent, or absorbed by the medical therapeutic model. It just depends on where the majority of the profession wants it to go.

Are there any other comments you'd like to share about the wonders of chiropractic?

I'd like people to understand that chiropractic is more than just a way to make a living and even more than just a profession. It's really a way of looking at life and of expressing more life. That's how I see chiropractic and how I see my role in it.

Years from now when people look at your tombstone, what would you want them to read?

My name in Hebrew means "increasing faithfulness." I guess I would like people to read that I was faithful to my philosophy, faithful to my community, faithful to my family, faithful to my God, and that faithfulness increased throughout my life.

❧

Joe B. Strauss, D.C., FCSC, graduated from Columbia Institute of Chiropractic (now New York Chiropractic College) in 1967. From 1978-94, he was a professor at Pennsylvania College of Straight Chiropractic. He has served as editor of The Pivot Review, a chiropractic philosophical publication, since 1983.

Dr. Strauss has written and published 18 books, including "The Journey," "Chiropractic Philosophy," "The Pivot Review: 1984-1991" and "The Pivot Review: 1992-1997," "Case Management for Straight Chiropractors," "Refined by Fire: the Evolution of Straight Chiropractic," "Higher Ground," "Enhance Your Life Experience," "Practice Building for Straight Chiropractors," "Reggie: Making the Message Simple" (a biography of Reggie Gold), "The Green Book Commentaries," and "Still Higher Ground."

In 1992, Dr. Strauss was elected a Fellow of the College of Straight Chiropractic. He has lectured throughout the United States and overseas in Japan, New Zealand, and England on the subject of straight chiropractic. He resides with his wife, Iris, in Levittown, Pennsylvania, where he has maintained a large private "Box on the Wall" (where patients pay what they can on the "honor system") practice for more than 41 years.

Who could be so lucky?

Who comes to a lake for

water and sees the reflection

of moon.

Rumi